Girls Rock!
Just the Way We Are

Wise Teens Offer Tweens & Moms Advice on Healthy Body Image, Self-Esteem & Personal Empowerment

Compiled and edited by Lisa Miller

Collectively authored by the Girls Rock! Teen Mentors:
Katie Atkinson, Katherine Bandoroff, Jordan Barnhill, Hillary Bullock,
Jasmine French, Jenny Hafley, Abby Miller, Emily Miller,
Chauncey Morton, Ravon Radmard & Molly Gallagher Sykes

Professional Health Team includes:
Anne L. Edwards, Psy.D., Donna Foster, R.D.,
Joan Griffith, M.D. & Katrina Hood, M.D.

ACKNOWLEDGEMENTS

This book grew from a series of Girls Rock! community workshops for girls and moms, a grassroots effort made possible by generous volunteers. Since May 2004, teenage role models and professional health experts in Lexington, Kentucky have inspired families from across our state and from as far away as Ontario, Canada. My heartfelt thanks go to the entire Girls Rock! Team, past and present, for helping so many by demonstrating the strength and power of the feminine spirit.

Pediatricians Katrina Hood and Joan Griffith, Psychologist Anne Edwards, and Dietician Donna Foster are a few of the dedicated health experts known as the Girls Rock! Professional Health Team, and they have served as thoughtful consultants on this book. While their conversations with four of the eleven teen authors can be found at length in the transcripts section at the end of Section II, you will hear their wise, authoritative voices in excerpts concluding each teen chapter.

I am deeply grateful to my sister-in-law, Jennifer Miller, who captured the team at our best in many of the photos included, and who generously spent hours and hours integrating the text and layout for this book.

Girls Rock! Teen Mentor Hillary Bullock designed our terrific web page (which you can find at www.thecompassionatecommunity.com/girlsrock/).

My own mentors provided many invaluable suggestions: Rachel Belin, Gene Brockopp, and Toby Christensen. Many thanks to friends and family for constructive help with editing: Holly Bandoroff, Kristin Beers, Hillary Bullock, Susie Bullock, Anita Courtney, Katrina Hood, Shaun Love, Fran Morris Mandel, and Denise Patch. Holly Bandoroff and Penny Miller Harris generously provided the seed money that made it possible for us to print this first edition.

And to my husband Jonathan Miller, you win the award for Best Girls Rock! Man! Thank you for your enthusiasm, love, and assistance.

Lisa Miller

Compilation and editing by Lisa Miller.
Format and design by Lisa Miller and Jennifer Miller.

First Edition 2006

Distributed by Girls Rock, Inc., girlsrockky@aol.com.
Printed by Lulu, Inc.; additional copies available for sale at www.lulu.com.

None of the authors or editors will receive financial compensation for their efforts. 100% of our net proceeds will be used to fund future Girls Rock! projects and events.

CONTENTS

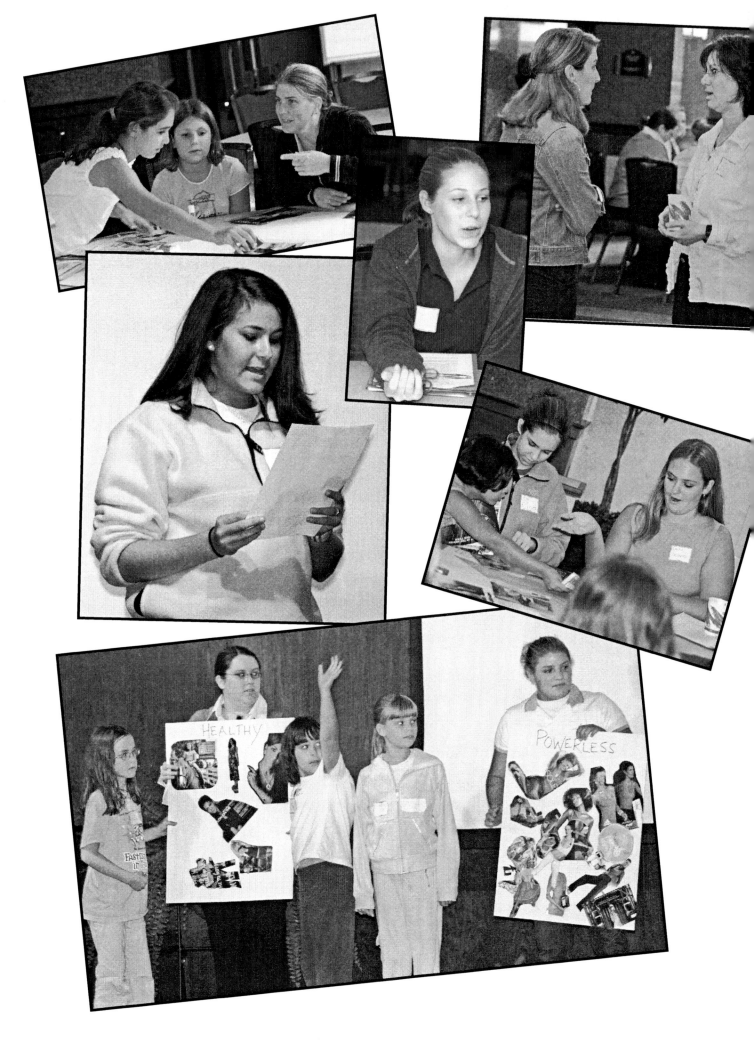

INTRODUCTION

Dear Moms,

What is your most heartfelt wish for your daughter? I believe that mothers everywhere long for their daughters to be spared the suffering they experienced. We hope and dream and pray that our daughters will not be detoured by messages and experiences that erode their confidence. We yearn for them to find their true callings and to live to their fullest potential as human beings. If we look at what have been the 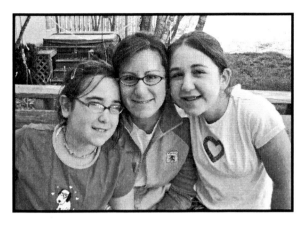 obstacles in our own paths, most of us have stories of internalizing messages early in life that we were somehow not okay. Imagine a world where our children are taught to celebrate and deeply cherish who they are through adolescence and into adulthood. This book can help you strengthen your relationship with your daughter and help her find the sure footing of deep self-esteem as she grows up, experiences new opportunities, and navigates social pressures as an independent woman.

Unfortunately, one unavoidable challenge comes from our culture's heavy focus on personal appearance. Just as mass media overwhelm women with advice on reaching a look that is unrealistic for most of us, it has become normal for our children to judge themselves and others harshly based on physical size, weight, and shape. Tragically, this is reflected in national statistics reporting that 81 percent of ten year-old girls are afraid of being fat, and half of girls between 12 and 14 say they are unhappy because they "feel" fat.[1] Many of us believe that we are acceptable only if we abide by the "be skinny" standard. This belief hangs on the demoralizing notion that self-worth is dependent on external standards.

While the numbers are heartbreaking, they reflect a devastating truth. In North America, the narrow standard of beauty that we have accepted is robbing our children of their birthright to be self-accepting beings whose authentic power resides internally. Media and advertising messages, peer pressure, the diet industry, and long standing family standards about weight, constantly reinforce the priority of thinness—the preferred look—over balanced nutrition and healthful choices, and over celebrating diversity and the inner spirit.

While tall, sleek, white women garner most of the attention in media-saturated North America, they actually represent only two percent of women born in this part of

---

[1] Statistics from the National Eating Disorders Association, available online (with academic research citations) at www.nationaleatingdisorders.org.

the world.[2] This means that 98 percent of us are shorter and less toned than the standard we obsessively pursue. How can our daughters love themselves when they are constantly assaulted by the message that their maturing bodies are unacceptable?

This zealous striving toward an unrealistic standard is causing unprecedented emotional damage in girls and women from early on. Reknowned body-image therapist and author, Kathy Kater, captures it best: "At a point in life when students should feel strong and confident in who they are, more and more of them feel there is something wrong with them. The impact of negative self-esteem and lack of confidence have long ranging effects into adulthood. Research shows that a growing child's inability to feel comfortable in their own skin can be detrimental in the formation of their identities."[3]

In the most abundant nation in the world, our girls are starving for a foundation of self-esteem that will support them through adulthood. How many truly self-accepting adult women with a positive body image do you know? Most of us have spent our whole lives loathing our genetically-programmed hips, cellulite, and bellies. Our girls are listening, and watching.

But there are solutions. We can inoculate our pre-pubescent girls and take an antidote ourselves. This book is a resource on which both you and your daughter can rely because it "shatters the lie that beauty is only skin deep",[4] and most uniquely, it is offered by youthful role models whom your daughters can relate to and emulate.

This book is written by teenage girls who have weathered their own storms, who have emerged with deeper self-esteem, and who want to help lead the way. They are extraordinary mentors because of their willingness to learn and grow from their experiences, and then to serve as role models and big sisters to their younger peers (our daughters). Known to tweens and moms in my community as the Girls Rock! Teen Mentors, they have facilitated healthy body image/self-esteem workshops for girls and moms since 2004.

Our grassroots, nonprofit organization, made up entirely of volunteers, is called Girls Rock! Self-Esteem, Healthy Body Image and Empowerment for Pre-Teen Girls and Moms. In day-long workshops, working side by side with professional health experts (pediatricians, a psychologist, nutritionists, spiritual leaders, a martial artist, and yoga instructors), these teen leaders reinforce the necessity of approaching health from a place of self-respect. They specialize in media literacy activities, but win popularity

[2] *Ibid.*

[3] Kathy Kater, *Healthy Body Image: Teaching Kids to Eat and Love Their Bodies Too,* page xiii (National Eating Disorders Association, 1998).

[4] Mind on the Media, www.mindonthemedia.org.

among girls and moms in attendance when they candidly describe their triumph over peer pressure and common adversity.

In addition to our teen mentoring approach, our excellent professional team brings diverse expertise as they serve as authoritative and accessible discussion leaders and presenters.

How To Use This Book

This book offers the wisdom that makes our Girls Rock! workshops so inspirational and useful for mothers and daughters. In their own voices, the teens' letters to you and your daughter serve to diffuse the "be skinny" oath which robs so many of us of emotional peace and true health. Knowing that young girls listen closely to older girls, these teen mentors offer practical advice focused on the development of inner strength.

Understanding and addressing these issues is vital for both you and your daughter. Based on personal experiences, and with guidance from health experts, each teen's chapter handles one crucial element of healthy development: the mother-daughter relationship, self-esteem, media literacy, triumph over challenges, diversity, self-acceptance, and an exploration of what "health" really means.

Most of the teen chapters (DEAR GIRLS AND MOMS) are intended for you and your daughter to read aloud together and then to discuss. This serves three key functions:

First, there is inherent strength in exploring these challenges as a team because you will share a framework for analyzing the messages about girls and women that bombard us daily.

Second, these initial discussions reinforce a vital habit of open communication between you and your daughter.

Third, reading together (and engaging in the fun, educational activities provided) deepens your bond as you share quality mom-daughter time at a critical period in your daughter's maturity.

Additionally, Section II includes some DEAR MOMS chapters for you to read privately for parenting purposes. Again, written by the best inside sources around, Section II is about prevention strategies. Topics include: disordered eating, communication with your daughter, seeking positive role models, advocating social causes, setting healthy boundaries, accepting your daughter's changing body, and living life from the spiritual core.

An afterword focuses on the hopes and dreams your daughter may have for her own children. It is for you and your daughter to read together.

I, too, am a mother of pre-adolescent girls. You can imagine my heart-break when my older daughter Emily (then nine) came home from school one Friday and announced, "I'm not eating this weekend because the girls at school want to be skinny." The Girls Rock! Mom-Daughter Workshops and this book are the results of my mission to help set things right for my daughter as she stood at the edge of a very dangerous cliff.

Today at nearly age 12, Emily is a leader among girls her age in the cause for self-acceptance and diversity. Part of the cure has come from continuously exposing her to positive role models who are happy and confident because of true inner power, and who are able to view life with greater perspective.

The rest of the cure has come from learning together, and then working as a mother-daughter team promoting healthy body image in our community together. More than ever before, my daughter sees me as a trusted ally, and as an empowered woman. This recognition is invaluable to Emily's healthy emotional and physical growth. I breathe a profound sigh of relief each time I acknowledge that my own kid is now okay.

So say to your daughter, "These are real girls just like you, in all shapes, sizes, and colors. They are content with themselves, and they are leaders because of this. They celebrate diversity, and they stand up for girls' rights to be diverse looking and thinking human beings. They remind us that we don't have to strive toward being skinny—just healthy and happy. All girls and women are beautiful, and we are all strong inside."

Perhaps while using this book, you too will connect more strongly to the part of yourself that is most wise, empowered, self-accepting, and enduring. We all need a support from time to time—especially since as adults we too are still affected by our diet-obsessed customs, often still holding out hope that someday we will be thin enough, pretty enough, and desirable enough—that we will finally start living when we fit into those pants. The truth is that we are already good enough, and already beautiful. And so are our daughters.

Sit down together and get comfortable—I know you'll enjoy this. It's nourishment for both of you, and you can always have more.

Peace, and best of wishes,

Lisa Miller
Mom, and founder of Girls Rock!

SECTION I

Dear Girls and Moms:

Dear Girls and Moms,

Read Section I of this book together, out loud! You'll enjoy your time together while learning about self-esteem and healthy body-image, and why they are so important for growing girls (and for moms who are already grown).

We are teenage girls ourselves (including two pre-teens), and we have written to you from our hearts about our experiences managing challenge, and about being happy and strong inside. Though our personal stories are all different, we share some things in common:

- We believe that girls everywhere are a part of one big sisterhood, and that we should support each other's differences.

- We know that there are a lot of messages in our culture about "being skinny", and that those messages are very damaging to girls and women.

- We feel that inner spirit is the most important aspect of every human being.

- We think about what "health" really means.

- We need to rely on our mothers for emotional support!

We suggest you read just a few chapters at time, relate your own experiences, and then give yourselves some time to let it all sink in before sitting down again to read the next few chapters. We have also included a few fun activities for you to do together from your place on your comfortable couch.

We are honored to be a part of your special mom-daughter time, and we know you will enjoy discussing the topics of this book together.

It's awesome to be a girl today! No matter what your age, we hope that you are excited about your place with us in this sisterhood, too.

Love from all of us,

The Girls Rock! Teen Mentors

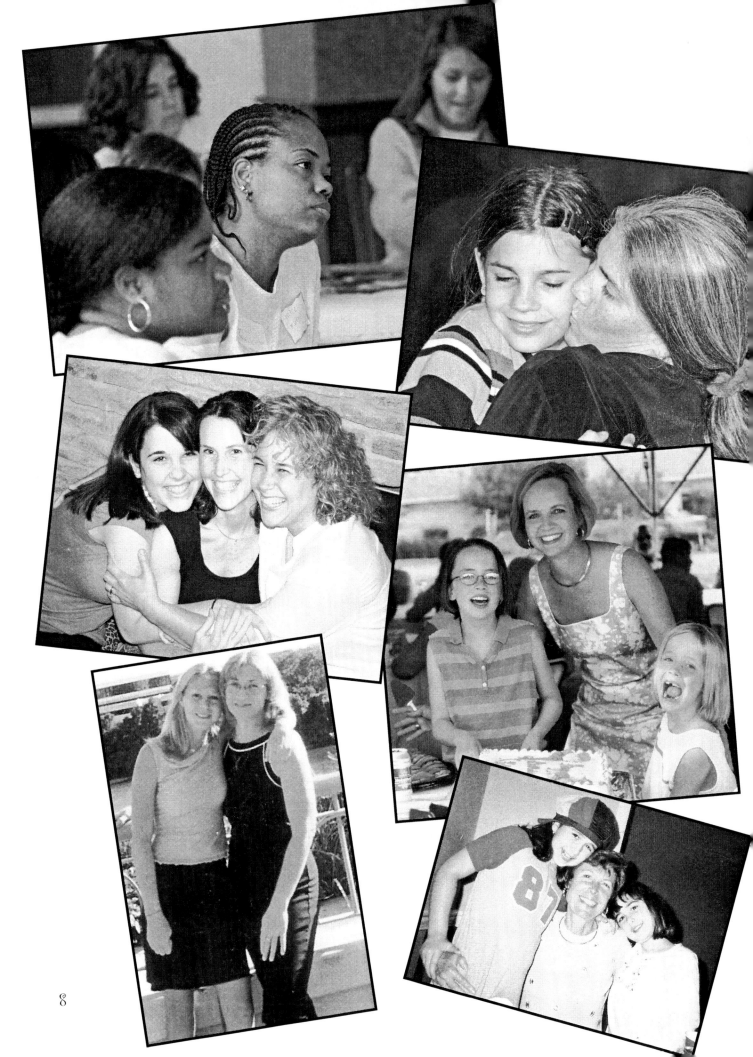

LEANING ON YOUR MOM
Jordan Barnhill, age 17

Dear Girls and Moms,

Our mothers would do anything in the world to help us be happy. They care about us unconditionally and love us no matter what. Your mom can be the best friend you will ever have.

It took me a while to realize that my mom actually knew what she was talking about. My advice is to listen to your mother and talk to her when you need someone. Our moms have been in the same positions that we are, and they have come out of their pre-teen years with knowledge and experience about how to live through it. Our moms can offer us strength that we didn't realize we needed.

It will help you and your mom to have an open and honest relationship, and that openness will make you a healthier person. It's not good for you to keep all your emotions bottled up inside. There are some things that you will not want to tell your friends. In those times, your mom will be there for you because she is a source of love, kindness, and strength that you can tap into whenever you need.

me, at age 9, with my mom

My mom has been here for me through all my celebrations and through countless challenges. When I was your age, she was always available when I needed a shoulder to cry on or someone to talk to. Now that I'm 17, she is still my shoulder to cry on.

After my fifth grade year at a private elementary school, my parents and I decided that it would be a good idea for me to try out a bigger, more diverse school. My old school was small and I knew every single person in my class. I thought it would be good to experience new people, new teachers, and a new environment.

Over the summer, my excitement grew with each passing day. The night before my first day, I couldn't sleep, and when morning finally came, I popped out of bed and got ready as quickly as possible.

However, as I left the house and began walking down to the bus stop, my stomach started to flip. The reality of the big change seemed to hit me all at once. Nervousness replaced my excitement and suddenly I wished that I could be anywhere else in the world except standing in front of the scary yellow bus. But, instead of running back into my mother's arms, I wiped my tears and put on a brave face for the beginning of a very long day.

All day, switching classes with three hundred other people in the hall was a lot scarier than I thought. I just barely made it through the day without an emotional breakdown.

Sitting on the bus ride home, I could feel the tears well up in my eyes. I searched down deep for the strength to hold them in until I was back in the safety of my own house. But spotting my mom out the bus window unleashed the flood-gates, and that night I cried in my mother's arms for at least two hours. I couldn't stop. I told her everything I was thinking, and about all my fears. I admitted that I was terrified that my new classmates would not like me and that I thought school was going to be so hard.

She let me get out everything I had pent up that day. She was like a sponge absorbing all of my sadness, pain, and anxiety. Her hugs erased all the day's bad memories, and her calm words eased my tension. No one else could have helped me that day except for my mother. I couldn't have unloaded this on my friends, teachers, or other relatives. I needed a special kind of nurturing. I felt that no one else could have listened to my fears, calmed my nerves, and loved me as much as she did. My mom filled me up with the confidence and strength I needed to be able to go back to school the next day. That night we talked until I fell asleep.

With time, I got used to my new school, made great friends, and earned straight A's the entire year. But, without my mom there for me that first night of sixth grade, I may have hid under the covers waiting for someone to rescue me. Instead, my mom empowered me to face my challenge with confidence. Knowing I would go home to her open arms helped me stay strong during the day.

For me, good friends are important, but there will never be anyone to fill my mother's shoes. Your mothers are there to do the same things for you. Tell them what you need and know that we all need our moms, even when we grow up.

Love,
Jordan

Q & A excerpt from our interviews with The Professional Health Team:

Girls Rock! **Teen**: Concerning your healthy body and healthy spirit approach, are there certain things you talk about with your own girls?

Dr. Hood: One of the biggest things we try to do, is focus on being a family that does things together—being together, playing together, going outside to kick a ball around. I try to spend time every night with each one of my kids before they go to bed. I just ask them questions about the day or about things they want to talk about. It is a special time for them and me. I think that is important. My oldest daughter and I are excited about a little mom-daughter overnight we're going to take before school starts to talk about some of the puberty issues that will soon be coming up for her.

"I'm So Fat, I Wish I Could Be As Skinny As You"
Emily Miller, age 11

Dear Girls and Moms,

Hi everyone. Two years ago in fourth grade, I went through a really hard time. Something was happening to the girls in my grade. The commercials and ads that we watched since we were little started to sink in. The message was that girls should be thin and glamorous, and that everyone should have a boyfriend. So we started complimenting each other on being "skinny" and criticizing ourselves on being "fat".

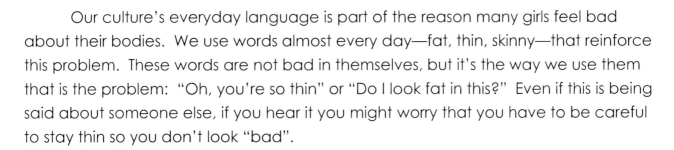

Body image is the way you think and feel about your body. It's what you believe you look like. When you always rely on other peoples' judgments of you, then you never feel content with who you are or what you look like. When your everyday language is about being skinny, your body image suffers. That's what happened to us.

Our culture's everyday language is part of the reason many girls feel bad about their bodies. We use words almost every day—fat, thin, skinny—that reinforce this problem. These words are not bad in themselves, but it's the way we use them that is the problem: "Oh, you're so thin" or "Do I look fat in this?" Even if this is being said about someone else, if you hear it you might worry that you have to be careful to stay thin so you don't look "bad".

Those words became a part of my everyday language and started changing my confidence about my own appearance. What I was hearing around me was meant to be innocent; but really, it hurt all us girls inside.

Soon, I thought that my belly was different from everyone else's. I was comparing myself to my friends. I didn't realize that everyone's entire bodies are different from one another, and I started thinking I was "fat". Even though my mom told me over and over again that I wasn't, it didn't help and I didn't believe she knew anything.

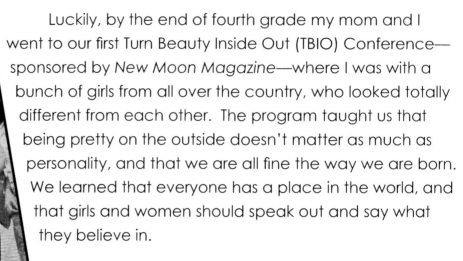

me, Jenny and Ravon
(we were presenters at the
2005 TBIO Conference)

Luckily, by the end of fourth grade my mom and I went to our first Turn Beauty Inside Out (TBIO) Conference—sponsored by *New Moon Magazine*—where I was with a bunch of girls from all over the country, who looked totally different from each other. The program taught us that being pretty on the outside doesn't matter as much as personality, and that we are all fine the way we are born. We learned that everyone has a place in the world, and that girls and women should speak out and say what they believe in.

This helped me change the way I was feeling about my body. I also realized something about being a girl: it's fun to get dressed up, paint your nails, go shopping, and try on shoes, but when it becomes an obsession, it's not good for us. It's great to be a girl, but we have to stand up for a deeper identity.

Being around the girls at this conference also helped me realize that trusting my mom was cool after all because they showed that they trusted their moms' opinions. My relationship with my mom really improved after that.

A lot of time has passed since then, and I have led healthy body image workshops for kids my own age. I even made a presentation at my second TBIO conference. The advice I'm about to give you is something I wish I had been told a long time ago. Make sure that when you are complimenting someone, it's because you think they are pretty and not because you wished you looked like them. If you do feel that you want to look like someone else, then you are judging yourself and comparing yourself to others, and this is not the best thing for you. It's not what's on the outside that counts, it's your inside.

Think about it, you like your friends because of their characteristics, not what they look like. They might be funny, fun to be with, and have the same interests as you, but hopefully you are not friends with them just because they are nice looking. Usually, good people that you'll meet in life won't care if you are the most beautiful or not. So don't go looking for that in others.

Some people really believe that telling someone that they are thin is a compliment, but you are hurting the person you are complimenting because it might make them worry that if they change, they won't be complimented anymore. I've learned that it's better to compliment people on their personality or what you like about them rather than their looks. And if you do want to compliment them on their looks, just say, "You are pretty!"

So remember, talking about being fat or thin just makes things worse for everyone. Next time you have a conversation, try to realize that language has a lot to do with problems girls have with weight, body image, and the way we think about ourselves.

It's sad that, today in sixth grade, some of the girls are still affected by the messages of our everyday language. I wish I could help those girls who worry about being fat. But there are some strong girls like me who have confidence in who they are and who have a healthy body image.

You are pretty just the way you are too; don't let language affect you too much.

Love,

Emily

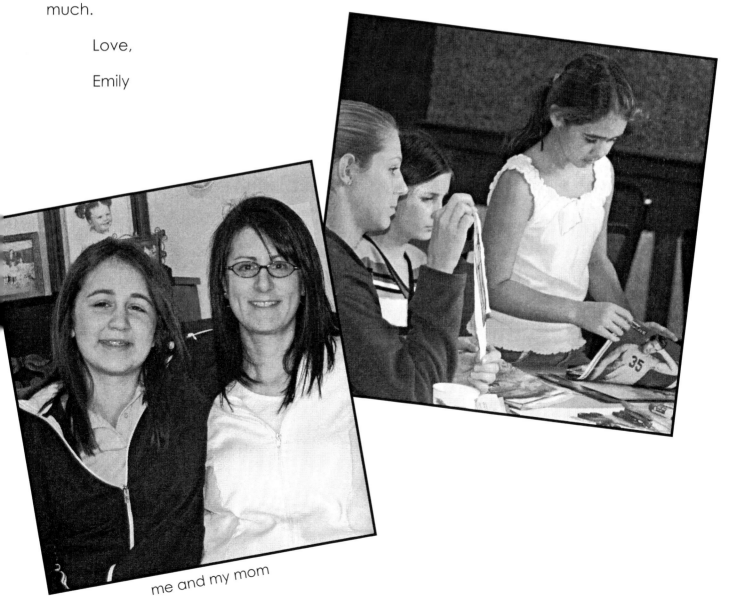

me and my mom

Q & A excerpt from our interviews
with The Professional Health Team:

Girls Rock! **Teen**: We hear the word "skinny" a lot in our culture, and a lot of time it is used as a compliment. What do you think about this?

Donna: I don't see that it is appropriate in any circumstance for someone to compliment with, "you are so skinny." That is labeling. I believe that it's inappropriate for anybody to comment on your body, or my body. It's a boundary violation. They're crossing over into something that they should not be making comments about.

Girls Rock! **Teen**: So what could be an alternative?

Donna: "You look beautiful in that color," or "you look great today, really put together." "Looks like you feel good, or have good energy." Or "that outfit is so flattering on you." But not about size, what gives another person the right to comment on size? If someone says something to me about my body — and it doesn't happen anymore, but it used to — I feel invaded, scrutinized.

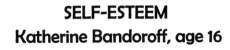

SELF-ESTEEM
Katherine Bandoroff, age 16

Dear Girls and Moms,

I think that self-esteem is feeling good about yourself and having confidence in what you do. Confidence and self-esteem are extremely important for happiness and success. There is no way you can accomplish anything meaningful if you do not believe in yourself.

My self-esteem originated from within my family and has helped me to believe in myself. My parents have always supported everything that I have committed to and dreamed of doing. They have taught me that attitude is everything and that without a positive attitude, nothing can go the way you want it to.

With their help, I have developed a very good attitude about life in general, and I carry that forward into my confidence. As long as I can remember, I have always had confidence in myself, and I feel that this is one of my strengths. This helps me do well in school and athletics.

Also, working hard to achieve my goals has made me successful. Once you accomplish a little, you can remember your achievement later during challenging times. This will help make you strong enough to work through obstacles.

I have definitely had my self-esteem challenged—but I worked through it at the end of a soccer tryout. Two years ago when I was thirteen, my coach came over to me and said that if I wanted to play on the better team, I would probably have to lose some weight. She was trying to let me know that coaches use a player's appearance to roughly scout them, and that they assume that someone like me who is not tiny—but big, muscular, and strong—doesn't have much speed. She was trying to help, but it was very upsetting and really hurt me.

Fortunately, my mom helped me a lot in this situation. We

me at age 11

spent the whole car ride home talking about it. She told me not to let it get to me, and to keep playing as hard as I usually do because that has already gotten me this far.   Not only did she ease my feelings, but she also made me feel good about the type of person I am—loving, caring, and unselfish. She reminded me that these traits alone would get me far in life.

I knew that I was a capable player despite the coach's warning about my weight. I love soccer and I play it all the time—it's very important to me. If my parents are ever looking for me, they can usually find me on the soccer field or in the backyard playing around.

Even though I felt bad, I bounced back the next weekend and played really well in my game. And, I played well through the season and became a leader on the team. I realized that I am good the way I am, and it doesn't matter what I look like.

Eventually, I put the hurtful experience behind me.   No one's looks should be an issue when they are playing soccer or doing anything else.

I hope you learn from my experience that no matter what other peoples' opinions, you should keep doing things you love, and self-esteem will come from it.

Katherine

Q & A excerpt from our interviews with The Professional Health Team:

Girls Rock! **Teen**: Why is self-esteem important to empowerment in girls?

Dr. Anne: Self-esteem leads to empowerment because it is so hard to feel a sense of competence, motivation, and to take initiative without healthy self-esteem. It seems like a cycle, that if you feel good about yourself, you feel more capable to explore your interests and succeed at them, which lead to you feeling good about yourself. Early on, if you get in a negative cycle of feeling you are not going to succeed or not good enough to do something, it leads you to miss opportunities to show yourself that you are good at things. Sometimes you have to take chances, even if you don't think you'll succeed. You will likely feel proud that you tried, even if you aren't great at it.

MEDIA LITERACY
Hillary Bullock, age 17

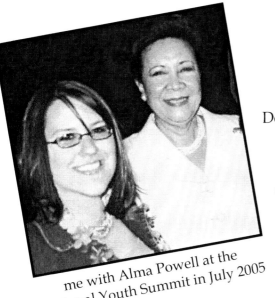

me with Alma Powell at the National Youth Summit in July 2005

Dear Girls and Moms,

Question: How should you deal with the media's distorted images of beauty?

Answer: Education. Knowing that the images of women on TV, movies, magazines, and the Internet don't really reflect what most of us look like, is a start. Media literacy means you can understand and analyze the messages that the media puts out there. Teach everyone in your life to know that the images of women in magazines, on TV, and in movies are not real. Those women look very different in real life.

In our culture, girls and women are put under a magnifying glass. Professional photographers, movie agents, and makeup artists have the job of making models, actresses, and musicians look picture perfect. The photos you see in popular media have been touched up and doctored using a process called airbrushing to make the women look stick-thin and blemish-free. What type of model do you see most in magazines? Most of them have similar bodies and looks, don't they? Our culture sells one type of look most often.

I want to see more accurate versions of beauty on TV and billboards—girls and women of all sizes, shapes, and colors, whose bodies aren't technologically altered to sell diet food or the latest fashion.

Also, when we look at glamorous Hollywood, the celebrities are at their best because they know people will be taking pictures of them. I hope you realize that those are special occasions and the celebrities don't wake up looking glamorous. They have bad hair days, just like you and me.

It makes me mad that many girls and women look at beautiful magazine covers and then feel bad about their personal "flaws." Everyone—different races, ethnicities, and sizes—should be celebrated in the media so that we can all feel naturally beautiful and represented and celebrated.

There is another problem with how the media tends to portray female celebrities. In photographs taken without permission, the women are captured during times when they would rather have privacy. Some photographers and magazines then exploit those private moments that highlight their human flaws in a way that causes us, the reader,

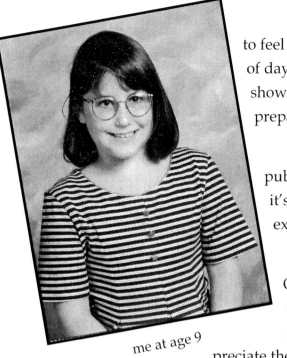

me at age 9

to feel ashamed and embarrassed when we have those kinds of days. It seems that all we see are extremes. Either they're showing up to awards shows looking perfect after hours of preparation, or they are exploited on a bad day.

I don't see much middle ground. Media outlets publish what consumers will buy—and for many people, it's probably more entertaining to look at photos that are extreme.

Of course, this is not to say that all media is bad. Our Girls Rock! team loves some television, movies, magazines, and popular music. We believe that the key is to enjoy these things in moderation and to appreciate them for what they are. Go ahead and let yourself be entertained! Just be sure to analyze the messages you are getting from your sources of entertainment. Don't fall into the trap of internalizing all those messages. In other words: Recognize and analyze, don't internalize. See page 19 for a fun mother-daughter activity that will make you more aware of these patterns.

So, I hope this is helpful. Media literacy is key! By knowing that what we see in the media is not completely real, and, by analyzing those messages, we have valuable tools in dealing with the pressure to fit into this unrealistic beauty standard. Reminding yourself of this truth will help you to not compare yourself to the inaccurate images all around you.

Love,

Hillary

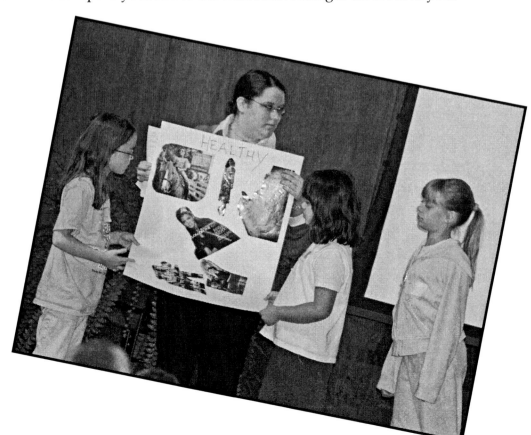

P.S. I really want girls and moms to become wise about the messages we all get from the media in our culture, so here is an easy activity for you do together. Pick up a magazine, tear out some of the ads of women, and answer the following questions together.

MESSAGES MATTER

Recognize: Sometimes women are made to look powerless in the situations they are in.

Analyze by asking yourselves… Is the woman in the ad in a situation that's unnatural or dangerous? Is her body in an uncomfortable position? Is she wearing clothes that are appropriate for the environment she is in?

Consider… It's normal for females to wear clothes that fit and flatter our bodies. However, would you wear a bathing suit to the bookstore, or only underwear out to dinner with friends, or a fancy dress to the gym? NO! If she is in an uncomfortable situation but smiling, her power as someone who takes care of herself properly is lessened. Think about the context of the situation when deciding if a woman looks healthy or powerless.

Recognize: Sometimes women are objectified in ads. (That means that they are being used and disrespected.)

Analyze by asking yourselves… Is only a portion of the woman's body being used in the ad? Is the woman smaller than the thing she is selling? Why might viewers think she is less of a person?

Consider… Especially when photos don't include a woman's head, it becomes easy to ignore her uniqueness, originality, and the fact that she is a human being with depth. Using only a portion of her body suggests that the model is not a whole person. This is often objectifying and demoralizing.

Recognize: Our culture focuses so much on beauty that we have come to believe that beauty = power. But this is not authentic power because external beauty is only one tiny part of who you are as a whole being.

Analyze by asking yourselves… Does the ad connect the idea of a beautiful face and body with power? If so, what might happen to the model's self-esteem when she gets older and her body and face age? Also, do our minds and spirits have anything to do with true beauty?

Consider… Humans are made up of body, mind, and spirit. Beauty, power, and self-esteem cannot be based solely on appearance because we are so much more than just that—we each have a soul and a purpose for being alive. We are more than our bodies. And, as we age, our appearance does change—it is inevitable and it is normal!

WISDOM IS POWER!

Q & A excerpt from our interviews
with The Professional Health Team:

Girls Rock! **Teen**: How can parents send a positive message of health and nutrition to their girls in a diet obsessed culture?

Dr. Anne: Parents can help by communicating with their daughters how they have been impacted by the culture themselves, because we all have, and how they fight getting sucked into it. (Diets they have tried and the focus they have had on appearance and how now they are trying to simply eat healthy, balanced foods and focus more on other things.) They can connect with their girls by sharing this.

They can also make it a mission to fight the culture together. In the *Girls Rock!* workshops, I suggest to girls and moms to have some kind of code word that they can refer to when something catches their attention about negative eating or body image messages. For example, if a relative comments on your weight and you don't feel comfortable addressing it directly, you can look at your mom and use the code word to acknowledge that both of you know the comment is inappropriate and that you will discuss it later. The same word can be used when watching an offensive commercial or when walking by magazines in the grocery store.

Girls Rock! **Teen**: How can parents reinforce a positive self-image in their growing girls?

Dr. Anne: It is a difficult job, and parents are not supported by our society. You have to seek out support to fight the cultural messages and instill healthy ideas in your daughter about her weight, eating, her body, and what is important in her life. The most important thing for you to do is to be a good role model. You must practice what you preach. If you are struggling, as these issues do impact all of us, helping yourself will be the best thing you can do for your daughter.

DIVERSITY, STRENGTH
Chauncey Morton, age 15

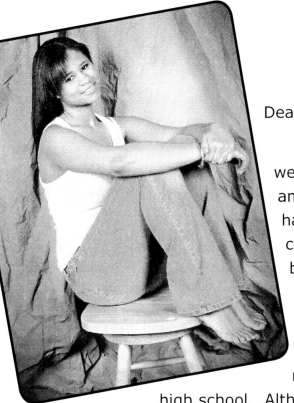

Dear Girls and Moms,

No two people are the same, so why should we all strive to look the same and be the same? I am African-American and will never have blonde hair and blue eyes unless I dye my hair and get colored contacts. If I were to do that, I wouldn't be the true me.

For most of my life I have lived in a pre-dominately white neighborhood and have gone to predominately white schools. There wasn't much diversity at all until I reached middle and high school. Although I always knew that being African-American made me "different" from my white friends, I never felt different—just content to have good friends and be part of the group.

But I remember the day I realized that I was differ-ent from all the other kids in my class—that I really was the only black girl. I was in the third grade and a class-mate, a white boy, called me a nigger. At the time I didn't understand the word so I wasn't hurt, but after I spoke to my parents about it I found out that it was a very degrading term for African-Americans. It is a term used to say that a black person is less than human.

me at age 10

My parents and principal got involved and the boy was suspended. My parents helped me realize that it wasn't okay for a person to call another human being such a degrading name. It taught me to take racism seriously and made me grow up faster because racism is a big issue. Every single person is a human being and should be respected by other human beings.

The sad part is that before the incident, I felt secure about myself at school and with my friends, then suddenly I felt set apart from the rest of my class and I began to struggle with the fact that I was not like everyone else. Because of being called that name, I felt like something was wrong with me. I asked myself, " If I'm not like them, am I going to be okay?" My parents had to really help me understand that I was not the name I was called.

It took me years to feel completely accepting of myself—even with my own group of friends who liked me the way I was. I would sometimes worry about little things that made me different from them, like my hair not being straight enough and my honey-colored skin getting so much darker in the summer.

Finally, by the end of my middle school years, I started to accept myself and become proud of my differences from others. I realized that so much diversity exists between people even in the same race, and no two people are exactly the same. African-Americans are light skinned people as well as really dark skinned people. If a whole race can be so many different shades, then it's okay for the world to be that way—and, even more, for me to be that way.

When I look back on that time in my life, I reach out for the little girl that I was and feel sorry for her because she had to go through all that insecurity at such a young age. But like my pastor said in church the other day: no matter how many obstacles you must overcome in life, they will build you up to be a person of strength. I'm an example of this. Even though I struggled, I feel good about myself now and I can be a mentor to you because of my experience.

If your skin, religion, body, or background is different from your friends, don't be ashamed. Be proud of yourself exactly the way you are. Learn from my story that you can overcome obstacles in your life, even when you think you can't.

Also, be sure to tell your parents and your school about any racist or generally negative comments aimed at you or kids you know. Don't try to keep that hurt inside. You need support, help, and the realization that we need diversity in our world to make it a more advanced, interesting, and creative place.

I want to leave you with a piece of advice I once heard that has always stuck with me: "people weren't created differently to all look and act the same."

Love,
Chauncey

Q & A excerpt from our interviews with The Professional Health Team:

Girls Rock! **Teen**: What advice do you give to your own daughters about being open-minded to everyone's differences?

Dr. Hood: When my girls ask questions that relate to differences in skin color, body type, religion and others, I first explain that it is natural for us to notice differences. How we react to those differences is ultimately what makes the distinction between acceptance of that difference and prejudice.

SELF-RESPECT, RESISTING PEER PRESSURE, AND DOING THE RIGHT THING
Jenny Hafley, age 17

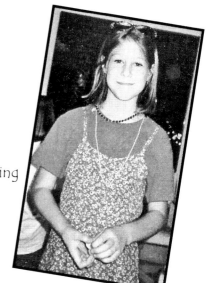

me at age 11

Dear Girls and Moms,

Peer pressure is when you feel like you have to do or say something because your friends think it is the cool thing to do. Being a person of integrity and self-respect is not about fitting a specific mold, but about creating an ideal for yourself and following it to achieve the things that are important to you. This will help you resist peer pressure. Know what your morals are and be true to yourself even when others may want you to behave in ways that go against what you believe is right.

There have been times when resisting the pressure to agree with others has been difficult, but I have felt that standing up for what I believe in is more important. When I was a camper at Camp Anytown, I was sitting in a small discussion group with other campers talking about discrimination within our schools. We had just talked about how important it is to choose our words wisely because we can say discriminatory things without even meaning to. (Discrimination is when a person is treated differently because of the things that make them unique, such as their age, skin color, religion, size, or background. It is a negative thing because it can be very hurtful and does not allow everyone to have an equal chance.)

Soon after this discussion, one of the guys in my group described something as "so gay". Even though this was the perfect time to point out that he had been discriminating in his language, I feared that it would not be the "cool" thing to do.

I decided to go ahead and say something to him because I knew it was the right thing to do, and I thought about how calmly I would say it in order to get my point my across. I explained it was not a good idea to use the word "gay" to negatively describe something because it is unkind to gay people, does not make sense, and his use of the word was not even describing homosexuality.

At first, he was defensive and told me that he had not really meant it the way I had taken it, and that everyone else knew what he meant. Although he did not agree with me at that very moment, I saw a change in his vocabulary as the week went on. After that, people in our group became more aware of their language and called each other out when something hurtful or disrespectful was said.

This situation gave me the confidence to leave the safe environment of camp and stand up for what I knew was right when I returned home. Today, when my friends tell jokes about someone's skin color, body type, or religion, I let them know that even though they are just trying to be funny, their humor is hurtful, inappropriate and discriminatory. When I point out that their choice of words could hurt someone's feelings, they usually wish they had not said it. But even if they don't stop, I still feel good knowing that I stood up for something I know is really the right thing to do, the moral thing to do.

Usually, peer pressure doesn't come from enemies, but from friends. This makes it even harder to say "no" to something you know you shouldn't try or agree with.   It is important that you set limits and stand your ground because you will feel much better about yourself in the end if you make the choice that leads you to do the right thing instead of giving in to peer pressure to be "cool".

When I was your age, I felt pressured to try things I did not want to try, and it forced me to make decisions that I knew were best for me. Sometimes kids think about smoking a cigarette or even drinking alcohol. When these suggestions are made by other kids, it can feel like extreme pressure. You really, really have to resist these kinds of pressures because if you give in to them, you could hurt yourself or get into a lot of trouble.

I want good things for you. Although it may seem cool, doing things like smoking and drinking are not good choices for someone your age. Don't even try that stuff. The deeper your respect for yourself, the easier it will be to know what you need to say "no" to.

As a person of integrity and self-respect, have things in your life that are important to you like: friends and family, your education, your sport, community service projects, art and music, animals, or any cause that you are passionate about. If you don't know what positive things are out there for you to become involved in, ask your parents and your teachers at school to help you figure it out.

You can be anything you want to be as long as you respect yourself and respect those around you. Peer pressure can be a hard thing to guard yourself against, but the more you stand up for your values, the stronger and more self-confident a young woman you will become.

Your Friend,
Jenny

Q & A excerpt from our interviews with The Professional Health Team:

Girls Rock! **Teen**: How does peer pressure make us vulnerable to the influence of others?

Dr. Anne: Peer pressure is a typical part of growing up. Everyone wants to be liked and to fit in. As we mature, we try to figure out who we are and where we belong. This uncertainty leaves us vulnerable to others' influence. Others try to influence us to find their place in the world as well. When we are influenced to do things that don't feel good to us, we may be giving in to peer pressure.

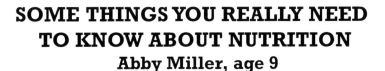

SOME THINGS YOU REALLY NEED TO KNOW ABOUT NUTRITION
Abby Miller, age 9

Dear Girls and Moms,

When you hear people talk about nutrition, you usually hear about calcium for bones, and eating more vegetables and stuff. But when I talk about it, I talk about other things that are pretty important to help you be healthy.

First, let's talk about labels. Labels are on most foods and they tell exactly what's in the food you are going to eat. When you look at a label, the first thing you read about is the serving size. This should be first because you want to know how much is enough. For example, on a bag of baked chips the serving size says 1 oz (ounce) (about 12 chips). So if you have more than that, then you are eating more than just one serving.

If you are eating granola, trail mix, ice cream, or stuff like that, you can use a measuring cup to measure the serving size that is enough—maybe it's 1/3 of a cup or 1/2 of a cup. After you measure it, put it in a bowl and eat it.

When you look at a label, have you ever noticed the column that says "saturated fat"? Well, saturated fat is a.k.a. lard! And lard is not something you want in your arteries because your heart can't work very well. So, if you see saturated fat, you can know that you shouldn't eat a lot of it all at once or all the time.

Next I want to talk about sugar. When you look at a label, check to see how much sugar there is. A little sugar is okay, but having too much in one serving isn't good for you because it makes you have a lot of energy quickly but then it makes you plummet down and get very tired. And it is something a lot of people are addicted to. Try not to have it in the morning because then you will crave it all day long.

So are you wondering how much sugar is enough? Usually at my house or the grocery store, if I want something sweet (that isn't a fruit), I choose something that has 12g (that means 12 grams) of sugar in it or less. If there isn't a label on something that we baked, I eat one or two servings for the whole day. That is enough. (By the way, 1 teaspoon of sugar = 4 grams)

Next, I want to talk about protein. It is one of the biggest things that you need for your body because it gives you energy. But this energy is different from the energy you get from sugar. Protein is like fuel for your car and lets you go for a long period of time instead of making you tired and then crash, like sugar does. You need protein at every meal.

Have you ever heard that breakfast is the most important meal of the day? Well, whoever told you that was right! You need protein in your breakfast to fuel the beginning of your day or else you will get really sleepy at school and your brain won't work so well.

In the mornings, I like to eat peanut butter or almond butter on toast (it's usually whole grain toast), or lox on toast with cream cheese (lox is smoked salmon), or eggs and turkey bacon, or sometimes oatmeal.

Now is the part about fiber. Fiber is important because it helps you poop.

Some people think that "poop" is a bad word but it's not because everybody has it. Fiber moves food through your body so that whatever your body doesn't use can get out of you (this is the waste). If you don't eat enough food with fiber in it, then your stomach will hurt because it is constipated. Foods you can eat with fiber are fruits, whole grains (bread, or oatmeal and stuff like that), vegetables, and nuts.

We have to talk about water. I drink lots of it because my body needs it. Our bodies are made up of 75% water, so you need to bring in lots of water to keep the water inside you from drying up. If you go a few days without water, you could really get sick and even die. I hardly ever drink juice or soda because it's loaded with sugar and I try to save my sugar for other things that taste better, like a brownie or cookie.

Last, I will talk to you about being hungry. If you eat when you are not hungry, then you are not listening to your body, but if you don't eat when you are hungry, then you aren't listening to your body either. Sometimes people want to eat when they are bored. This is not too good because eating is for being hungry.

You know you are hungry when your tummy starts to get that empty feeling, or when it grumbles. If you don't give yourself food at those times, you might start to get that dizzy, sick feeling. Just listen to your body.

So now that you know more about nutrition, why not go ahead and try some of the things I just told you about? Knowing all of this will make you smarter and healthier!

Love,

Abby

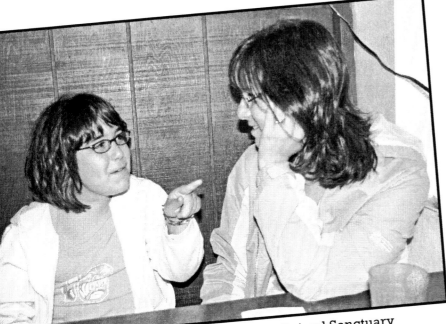
me and my mom at the Best Friends Animal Sanctuary

**Q & A excerpt from our interviews
with The Professional Health Team:**

Girls Rock! **Teen**: So where is the line crossed by a parent who wants their child to eat healthy but who is afraid of their child becoming 'fat' or overweight?

Donna: The line is crossed when the amount of time and attention becomes more than it should be, and when it's really emphasized, and that's the only thing the child hears. It's a balance. It's normal for bodies to change throughout a person's lifetime, and if parents are okay with their bodies, their children will see that.

Girls Rock! **Teen**: So how can moms teach their daughters to love themselves physically?

Donna: By loving themselves first. And then it's automatically passed down.

SELF-ACCEPTANCE
Katie Atkinson, age 16

Dear Girls and Moms,

I completely accept myself the way I am. I was born without a left arm. This has never, ever been an excuse not to do things. When I was little, my parents wanted me to learn how to be independent so that when I got older—the age I am now—I could do things for myself. I learned to tie my shoes and wash dishes just like everyone else. I don't give up just because something is hard. I know that I have impressed people with how hard I work. If I can't do something, I get really determined to learn how.

me at age 10

I never felt self-conscious about my arm until 9th grade when my dance coach told me that she didn't want me to dance at a competition that was the very next day. We had been practicing for months and the entire team was ready. She gave no clear explanation at the time, but we all knew it was because of my arm.

This was extremely upsetting and it made me feel really bad about myself. It was one of the first times anyone had treated me differently because of my arm, and it made me wonder about myself and about whether I was capable.

Of course my parents got involved and they were very supportive of me. But I was shaken up for a while because I realized that there are some people out there who will put you down and say you aren't good enough.

Eventually, time passed and my family and friends helped me a lot. I realized that I hadn't done anything wrong and that there wasn't anything "wrong" with me. It was just that I had a coach who was wrong.

This taught me that I should never let anyone make me feel bad about myself. I'm a strong and independent person, and confident in my body and in the way I present myself. I have learned that I don't have to look a certain way to be accepted.

The word confidence makes me think about all the stepping-stones I have taken to come to the point where I am now. I think about how much I've changed and how hard I've worked to become an independent person, to like myself, and to feel good. Confidence and self-acceptance come from your experiences.

I feel that self-acceptance is one of the most important things we learn as we grow up. It means loving yourself the way you are and being happy with who you are. Everyone has specific areas they are insecure about. You shouldn't worry about your imperfections because everybody has them. No one is perfect and that is something I would like you to remember. I don't want you to worry about what other people think about you. It doesn't matter what others think. We are all born with the capability to accept ourselves. It's up to each one us to chose whether or not to do so.

Definitely surround yourself with friends who accept you for who you are, and who love and accept themselves too. It's very hard to feel peaceful and accepting of yourself if others around you are constantly self-critical; this could really make you over-analyze your own "flaws".

Don't forget that talking to your mom can really help if you are having trouble accepting yourself. Your mom has been in your position before and has already experienced what you're going through now. I have relied on my mom for a lot of help. She always gets me to see that the whole world isn't ending because of my problem, and that things are not as dramatic as I think. She tells me about what happened when she was in school, and we talk about how to handle difficult situations.

So be strong and always believe in yourself no matter what.

I hope that after reading this you will accept yourself more deeply, and if you don't, learn how by talking to your family and friends and read the *Chicken Soup for the Soul* books. Admire someone truly good like my 8th grade teacher who had a lot of light, cared about all of the students, and talked to us about strength and acceptance.

I'm so glad that I learned to accept myself because now I'm truly happy with who I am and who I have become. I learned that being unique isn't a bad thing and that, in many ways, it has made my life better and special.

You deserve to realize how wonderful you are, too.

Love,

Katie

Q & A excerpt from our interviews with The Professional Health Team:

Girls Rock! **Teen**: What lessons do you like to share with the girls and moms who attend Girls Rock! workshops?

Dr. Griffith: I would like to think that the most important message I can share is that it is important to maintain balance in one's life—physically, spiritually, mentally, and emotionally. Once we maintain that balance, then life is worth living and enjoying.

Girls Rock! **Teen**: How do you define beauty?

Dr. Griffith: Beauty is that quality of life that makes you feel as if all is right with the world.

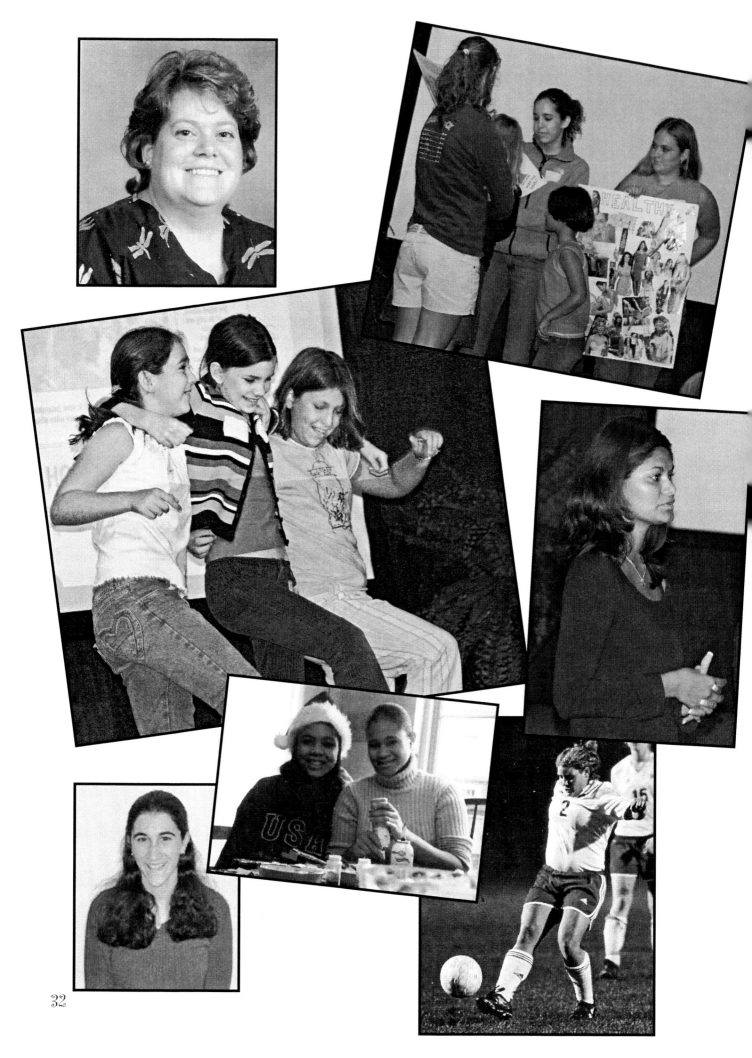

WHAT IS "HEALTHY"?
The Girls Rock! Teen Mentors

MOLLY, age 18:

Healthy is a state of contentedness in mind and body. It is not necessarily a life without hardship, but it is an ability to overcome hardships.

KATHERINE, age 16:

In my mind, a healthy human is someone who exercises, is a happy person who loves herself and others in her life, and who is mindful of what she eats but doesn't make food her life focus.

To maintain an overall healthy body image, you must be both physically and mentally healthy. Many people don't consider health as being anything other than physical wellness, but emotional health is also extremely important. Stress, depression, and unhappiness are all components of health. These can be helped by good exercise.

I love to sweat when I am working out or playing hard. It's important for the body because it excretes toxins and stress out of the body. After I am finished working, sweat is one way of measuring how hard I have worked. It makes me feel good about what I have just done with my body; I have just worked hard to keep it happy. I feel that if you are going to work hard, put forth as much effort as you can, so you do sweat a lot.

Last, making mistakes is healthy. Even though it is hard to watch yourself fail and it feels like your self-esteem is hurt, I find that failure is very important. No one wants it to happen all the time, but the few times it does happen, it really helps you learn from the previous mistakes. You can't improve aspects of your life if you can't figure out how they need to be adjusted.

CHAUNCEY, age 15:

Being healthy means being content with the person you are—being accepting of yourself.

JENNY, age 17:

To me, being healthy means living in a way that makes me feel good and function well physically, mentally, and spiritually. Eating foods that are good for me, and being physically active gives me energy and lets me focus on other things like school and friends.

JORDAN, age 17:

A full, healthy life is one that contains large amounts of passion. Once you have found something that you enjoy doing, keep on going because it will fill your life with happiness.

My passion is acting and always has been. I have loved performing ever since I was little. I love the rush of adrenaline that I get each time I'm about to go on stage, and I love the chance to step outside of myself for the few hours of each performance. It's my time to play.

It is so important for every girl to have an outlet for her energy—whether it is sports, theater, playing an instrument, or anything else—passion in something constructive is a foundation for health.

JASMINE, age 15:

Healthy is being mentally in shape and taking proper care of your body. It's about staying active and doing things you love—whatever you find interesting (for me it's sports and church groups). Health is about maintaining a good relationship with your mother.

KATIE, age 16:

Healthy is taking care of your body, exercising regularly, eating good foods, and finding a balance among all those things.

ABBY, age 9:

Being healthy is listening to what your body tells you it needs—like food, exercise, rest, and TLC!

RAVON, age 17:

I believe that health is more than just fitness and well-being. Health is more than just numbers on a scale, or a doctor's check-up, or a gym membership. Health is a balance among your body, your mind, and your spirit. It is understanding that you can eat broccoli and a candy bar, too!

Health is understanding that if you treat your body with respect, it will be a strong instrument for you to play soccer, or to learn to speak Spanish, or to play the trombone. It is about growth and maturity, and making wise decisions about what you put into your body, and about how you treat it. Health is the promise and the product. If you promise to continue to take care of yourself and set a healthy example for others, your body, your mind, and your spirit will repay you with health and a long happy life.

Health is like breathing; you can't live without it.

EMILY, age 11:

Healthy means taking care of your body in the way you know is right. It is exercising, eating healthy food, and most of all, having fun. Talking and expressing your feelings is healthy and normal. And don't forget, laughter is really good for you!

HILLARY, age 17:

For me these days, health is so much about letting people into my life who love, support, and want the very best for me. It's learning how to do more constructive things for myself that I'm not always comfortable with—for example, asking for a listening ear or a shoulder to cry on when things don't go as planned, or walking for an extra 30 minutes. Health is doing the things I need to do, even if they're not what I'm used to doing.

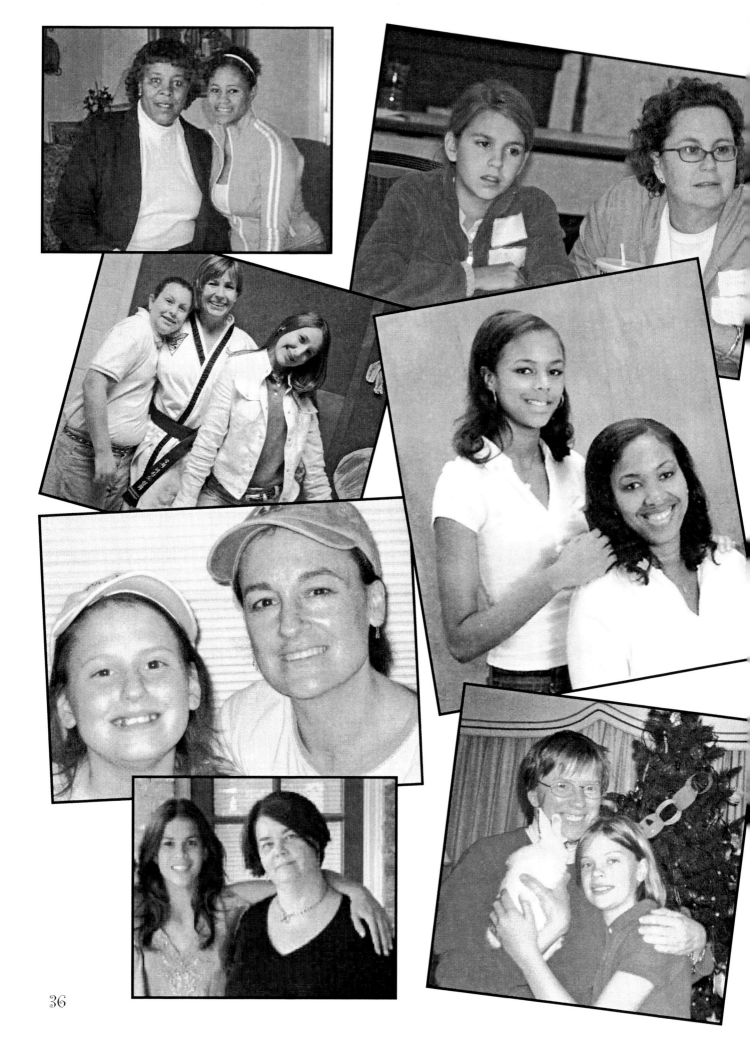

"WHAT I SEE IN YOU" ACTIVITY

It is wonderful when we are reflected from someone's loving eyes. It is also helpful because it reminds us of our unique, genuine inner qualities.

Using the following format as a guide, find paper for each of you to write on. At the top of your separate pages write: What I See In You. Now, write to each other from your hearts about the special qualities you appreciate in one another. Turn the page to see one possible format.

Need a little help getting started? Consider some of these descriptive words and phrases:

courage   Light   talent   an athlete

insightful   **a bright spirit**

a teacher

intelligence   **someone who doesn't give up**

an animal lover

a sensitive soul   peace

sunshine   a healthy person

someone who takes good   a love of God
care of herself and others

generous   **a nature lover**

passionate   a kind heart   someone who loves me

a good student   a good citizen

an adventurer

strength   one who accepts others

an old soul

a good friend to others   kookiness

laughter   a lot of personality

an artist   beauty

a talented person   thoughtful

kind

an activist   a book lover   **a leader**

Dear Mom (if you are a mom, write, Dear Daughter),

In you I see

I love our time together because

When I think about you I feel

Love,

SECTION II

Dear Moms:

The following letters cover a range of topics for you to read privately for parenting purposes. Written by the best inside sources around—our healthy teens—this section is about prevention strategies and handles sensitive topics, including: disordered eating, communication with your daughter, seeking positive role models, advocating social causes, setting healthy boundaries, accepting your daughter's changing body, and living life from the spiritual core.

Please consult a professional in your community if you realize that you and your daughter would benefit from more support than this book can offer.

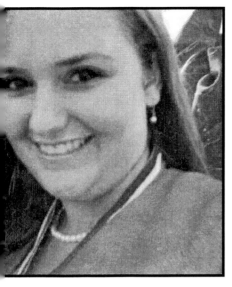

THE IMPORTANCE OF ACTIVISM AND
ROLE MODELS IN A GIRL'S LIFE
Ravon Radmard, age 17

Dear Moms,

Being involved in community service projects leaves me no time to mope in front of the mirror. It fosters relationships with people who share my similarities and respect my unique differences. For example, spending time with the other girls while working on this book has reinforced that the way I look and the numbers defining my body weight cannot stop me from achieving great things unless I let them. So many times I've heard that it's what's on the inside that counts more than the external. Guess what I've discovered—IT'S TRUE!

But activism is not just a distraction, it is deeply fulfilling. Much of my happiness comes from being involved in organizations that help others, and ongoing service projects provide me opportunities to meet people who are just as excited as I am about changing the world for the better. Here in Lexington, I'm involved in the Kentucky Conference for Community and Justice (KCCJ) as well as the Mayor's Youth Council.

A great reward for my service has been knowledge. I have learned a lot about equality and fairness for everyone—and about how racism, stereotyping, and discrimination affect our world. I know that the freedom to be happy and live a life of peace is an opportunity we are all born with that no one else has the right to take away.

This is very important to me, especially because of my multi-cultural family background. I believe that all human beings have rights that should not be violated. Fighting for justice has become one of my passions.

Also, through my community activism, I've learned invaluable leadership skills. Right now, I'm in the process of starting a club at my high school to help with national and international disasters, providing relief for families who have experienced loss.

I know you worry about negative influences on your daughter. I really believe that young girls benefit from having role models or mentors outside of the family. Though you are trying to instill confidence and empowerment in your daughter, having this reinforced from others will enhance and validate your effort. Role models can help ignite her interest and passion for the greater good—those things that are outside herself and her family, but that she is a part of.

The genuine relationships I've formed with my mentors and the bonds we've forged while working together on projects is invaluable. I cannot put a limit on the amount of confidence they've helped instill in me.

Through KCCJ, I met one of my mentors—a wonderful, caring woman named Mahjabeen Rafiuddin, who encourages me to be proud of myself and my background, and to be compassionate for others.

All of this has brought me to my role as a mentor and role model to younger girls today. I'm now passing it on. The sky is the limit for all the youth who are willing to give a little time and effort. The most important thing I've learned about myself is the power I have as a motivated girl. Self-acceptance, creating goals beyond the mirror, and the cause for justice are just the beginning for each one of us.

So I'm asking you moms, what is your daughter's emerging passion? She needs to find her niche—to realize that she is a participant in the world. You can even join a community cause together to help get her interested. Whatever it is, allow room for her ideas, goals, and motivation, and let her run with them. The feeling she gets from this will fill her with empowerment, and this will shine through everything else she sets out to accomplish.

Love,
Ravon

Q & A excerpt from our interviews with The Professional Health Team:

Girls Rock! **Teen**: Why do you feel it is so important that we help girls grow up into healthy and strong women?

Dr. Griffith: I think it's important that females realize that there is no better time than right now to be a female—to be energetic about life and the opportunities that avail—to be healthy and strong. I think health means that you have a positive attitude, even in the midst of trouble. It is important to be healthy in one's outlook so that you can survive the challenges of life.

Girls Rock! **Teen**: Is there anything I haven't covered that you would like girls, moms, and us teen mentors to know?

Dr. Griffith: Continue to try to find ways to help girls to realize it's okay to be female. As a matter of fact, it is exciting to be a female!

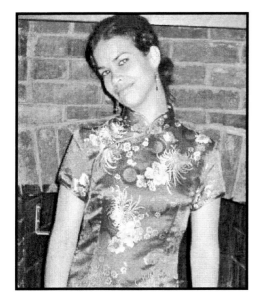

HELP AVOID AN EATING DISORDER NOW
Molly Gallagher Sykes, age 18

Dear Moms,

Isn't it funny? Even though you've likely had experiences similar to those of your daughter, you may feel powerless to help her now. When you tell her she is beautiful, she refutes it. When you try to talk to her, she closes her mouth tightly. When you struggle to put into words the wisdom you gained from your own teenage years, she has only five words for you: "It's not that easy, Mom."

Your daughter is right. It isn't that easy. And that is why she needs you. You have many doubts about whether you are doing the right thing. Even worse, you worry that your child's tiniest problems are your fault. They doubt, and you doubt. When it comes down to it, you must take the leadership role in guiding your daughter away from doubt and give her the ability to fight doubt—even without you by her side. There are many good resources for you to consult as you prepare to be your daughter's mentor—her compass in the storm.

I am not a mother. In fact, I'm only eighteen, which is a long way from reaching the experience and wisdom that you have. However, I may be able to give you a little advice on how to help your daughter because I have only recently gone through the years of adolescence, and the hardships and lessons are still fresh in my mind.

Additionally, I have a special perspective because I am in remission from anorexia nervosa—an eating disorder characterized by excessive exercise and restricting of food. I was diagnosed with this disorder in my eighth grade year at about the age of 14. It is a disorder that I will forever have, though I am healthy at this time.

Because of this eating disorder, I know all too well the pressures of society and how those pressures can distort the mind of even the most strong-willed and independent girl. I remember that in fifth and sixth grade, I had little or no regard for what was 'cool' and had never read an issue of *Seventeen* magazine. But just two years later, I was cutting my meals in half and posing in front of the mirror desperately trying to look like Britney Spears, a symbol of the ideal girl. Though I was a thin, slightly underweight girl, there were messages all around me that she was perfect and that I was not.

In our body-focused culture, the mind can become entirely illogical about things it hears. Accepting extremes for fact, ideas can become dogma. My mother, of course, did tell me I wasn't fat but it never reached me. I was already consumed by the obsessive voice of anxiety in my head that always had a great argument for continuing on my path of self-destruction.

I began to pull away from my family—becoming incredibly withdrawn and spending all my time alone in my room. I didn't want to eat with my family or go places where I might have to eat—so I didn't go out with my friends anymore either. I concentrated on perfection in my schoolwork so much that it became connected with being perfect in my body. I became very high-strung and moody.

This was a sudden change in my personality, but my parents regarded it as the normal feelings that teenage girls go through. They weren't aware that I was starving myself, and that because of it I was losing my hair, had stopped having my period, and was bruised all over from kidney exhaustion.

Luckily, my doctor discovered that I was in the negative percentile for weight, and told my mom to sign me up for counseling and a nutritionist.

It was only through talking to a nutritionist, from whom I learned how the body really uses food, and the terrible consequences of my starvation, that I began to take my problem seriously. With the joint help of this nutritionist and a psychotherapist, I eventually acknowledged that the arguing voice in my head was an eating disorder—that I had a disease which distorted my body when I looked in the mirror—my reflection ceased to be the real me.

With a lot of help and effort, I've just recently graduated from intensive therapy with my nutritionist, and I'm getting ready to leave for college. I finally feel comfortable managing my nutrition on my own, though I must watch myself to ensure that I don't lose weight again.

You really need to know what your daughter is learning from all sources, and then talk about all of it—analyze and dissect that information about body image so that her mind doesn't become fixed on a belief about beauty and perfection. This requires you to know more about health—educate yourself by going online, finding a book, attending a Girls Rock! workshop, or making an appointment with a nutritionist so that everyone in the family can know what health and well-being is about.

A big part of my own healing came from setting up a support system between my mom and me. Her support is extremely valuable to me and I now rely on her for reality checks to help me defeat the eating disorder voice in my head that sometimes says, "you are ugly and fat." I had to learn to trust my mom on this when I was already in crisis, but you can set up this trust now while your daughter is young.

Today, my mother and I cherish our deeper relationship—one great thing that we do is mom-daughter lunches where we talk about everything from me to politics. Also, going for walks together is great because adding that physical movement to our talks has strong physiological benefits. Basically, we just like spending time together.

I feel it's so important that you initiate this kind of frequent, open communication with your daughter. You should always know how your daughter is managing her challenges and how she feels about things in her life.   This quality time will definitely help prevent feelings of doubt and pressure from overwhelming her. You don't have to solve her problems for her, but definitely be the shoulder to cry on.

Of course, not every kid develops an eating disorder. However, many girls today grow to become hypercritical of their bodies which leaves a constant trend of self-doubt. But you can and should help your daughter feel secure with her body. You may think that you don't have as much influence on your daughter as her friends and the media, but the truth is that you are the strongest, most powerful influence of all.

As your daughter's role model, it's very important that you avoid self-criticism in front of her. Talk about yourself in a loving way and leave out the talk about dieting. If you are on a diet and your daughter sees you becoming confident and excited about your weight loss, it can be tricky because she might feel encouraged to mimic you for weight loss and confidence, while sacrificing her nutritional needs. While taking good care of yourself, you must be careful not to focus too much on all of this.

In addition to your prevention efforts, there are a few other things I strongly recommend in preventing an eating disorder. One of these is consistent moderate exercise which sets up the body for the healthy cycle of using fuel appropriately and which helps to keep mood stable.

Another is monitoring whom your daughter is spending time with. Do her friends talk about dieting and being thin? You've got to analyze this with her to help determine whether her friends are helping her feel good about herself or not. It's better to feel a little insecure while trying to find new friends than to stay with safe friends who make her feel ashamed of her body.

When I was younger, my best friend told me that my "big butt" was the reason boys weren't interested in me—and that they liked her because she was "skinnier". I was actually a healthy, thin girl, but this affected me deeply, and I decided to try starving myself. This is an eating disorder trap for many, many girls. Diffuse this before it happens. Talk to your daughter now about the fact that people don't always say things that are true and that sometimes they have other agendas.

When I was in the recovery process, my therapists advised me to always engage myself in things I love to do as this would distract my mind from its general trend of worry and self-doubt. I found purpose through French Club, Key Club community service, and diversity training with the Lexington Youth Leadership Academy. Having my voice heard through the Mayor's Youth Council was rewarding and fulfilling.

Though I was reluctant to engage in these things, my mom was the one who pushed me to do them and once I started an activity, I realized it was fun and rewarding. My worries had been keeping me from experiencing life. I feel fortunate now that my mom took the right step in not letting me sit at home all day feeling sorry for myself.

There was a time I waited for the sun to rise and to set. I waited for days to pass with no goal in mind, and I didn't enjoy anything. I just waited for each day to be over. But now I really like to make the most of all the time I have. I have fun doing stuff and I forget what time it is and what I need to do tomorrow and what I did yesterday. It's a really good thing to live in the moment.

I hope that my story can help you mentor your daughter and serve as prevention. Being prepared can help you and your daughter avoid living my story in the future. Always make sure that you know your daughter. Don't let a day go by that you don't have a sweet conversation with her, even if it's something silly. Talking to your daughter lets her know she can always talk to you when she needs to.

With your help, your daughter can overcome doubt in her life. You can't always avoid problems or solve them, but you can create a safe place for her to go. Be her mentor, hero, and counselor. The quality time you spend together now and the secure woman that she becomes will make it all worthwhile.

Sincerely,

Molly Gallagher Sykes

Q & A excerpt from our interviews with The Professional Health Team:

Girls Rock! **Teen**: What is an eating disorder?

Donna: An eating disorder is any way that one uses food to manipulate weight, or a way a person copes with life in unnatural ways—denying hunger, eating when not hungry, any way that's manipulative of food.

Girls Rock! **Teen**: How do you feel about our culture's habit of weighing ourselves? How much should the numbers matter?

Donna: Not at all. The question is: How do you feel? Buy clothes that fit, that make you feel good! We don't need numbers. The more our culture is obsessed with thinness, and we have been, the bigger our population gets. And there is no acceptance of diversity in body sizes!

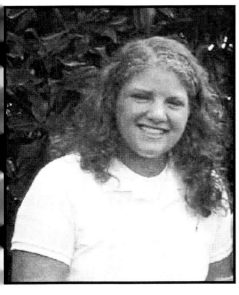

ACCEPTING YOUR DAUGHTER'S BODY THE WAY IT IS
Katherine Bandoroff, age 16

Dear Moms,

While your daughter is going through the process of pre-adolescence, it might be hard for both of you. It can be a challenge for you to see how grown up she is becoming; the teenage years approach parents very quickly.

Because girls are very sensitive at this age, one of the most important and helpful things you can do as a mother is to appreciate your daughter for who she is, rather than dwell on her body type, or on how it is changing. Of course you should talk to her about these changes, but don't dwell on them. Make sure to let her know she is great the way she is.

I have seen girls struggle because they were trying to please their mothers instead of just being happy with themselves. My mom and I have extremely different shapes—she is small and petite, and I have broad shoulders and a lot of muscle. However, these differences have always been okay.

Even though I look different from my mom, she understands that this is my body type and there is nothing that anyone can or should do to control that. She has never caused me to feel weird about my body type or tried to change me. My mom always tells me I look nice. (Although, she does hate it when I wear my hair up in a ponytail all the time. One time when she was driving me to a dance, even though I had my hair down, she noticed that I had my pony-tail holder around my wrist, and she pulled it off and threw it out the window!)

But most importantly, my mom loves me for who I am inside. As I said in the chapter on self-esteem, my confidence originated from within my family and has helped me to believe in myself. With my mom's help, I have developed a very good attitude.

Your daughter is who she is from the inside out. All the physical changes she goes through will never affect the person she is in her heart. It will help her a lot to know this.

Katherine

Q & A excerpt from our interviews
with The Professional Health Team:

Girls Rock! **Teen**: What is the one most important piece of advice you could give a mother about helping her daughter adjust to puberty?

Dr. Hood: I think that it is beautiful. So many girls are scared of it and they don't want to have the extra hair, the rolly tummies, the curvy thighs, and the bigger breasts. But all of that together makes you a woman. Seeing it as an opening of a window to the next part of your life is really exciting, and saying it's normal is important.

Also, having mothers talk to their daughters about what they went through and what they were concerned about would help. Talk about the different products you use for periods, so it's not embarrassing when it happens. It helps girls to be prepared if they happen to get their first period at school, so they aren't so scared. I believe that more knowledge is more power.

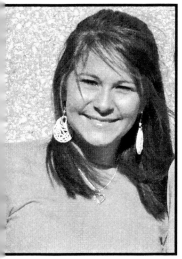

TRUST AND COMMUNICATION
WITH YOUR DAUGHTER
Jordan Barnhill, age 17

Dear Moms,

I am lucky to have such a wonderful mother. We have always been close with very good communication between us, and so I speak to you from this foundation.

I feel that one of the most important things you can do for your daughter is to maintain an open and honest relationship with her. That relationship will be a touchstone for her as she goes through the trials and tribulations of growing up. Establishing a good relationship with your daughter early on when she is young is key because if she grows up feeling comfortable and safe being honest with you, then she will have an easier time confiding in you about the serious stuff later on.

In building this relationship, be honest with your daughter. Sugarcoating or hiding the truth will not prepare her to cope. You can be truthful about the facts without scaring her. When I have a question, my mom answers it to the best of her ability. Whether it is what I want to hear or not, she gives me a real answer and helps me cope. For example, when your daughter comes to you and asks why she doesn't look like the cover girl on the magazine, be honest with her and help her see the big picture about the beauty myth. Don't tell her to ignore the magazine or that she should be happy the way she is. That answer is not realistic because it is impossible to ignore every single magazine cover, television show, and commercial. Instead, let your daughter express how those stereotypes make her feel. Talk about ways for her to cope with that pressure, instead of shutting it out.

I have felt that my mother's sincerity with me has allowed me to be honest with her. Even though an honest relationship with your daughter means being truthful about reality, you will sometimes have to hold back some of your feelings about what she tells you. If your daughter tells you something that upsets you or makes you angry, you might express that but make sure that you don't go overboard. Overreacting will scare her and may cause her to hesitate to confide in you in the future.

However, this does not mean that you should act like you are okay with everything that comes out of her mouth. I suggest giving your daughter advice to steer her in the right direction, but ultimately, you have to let her grow up and make some decisions for herself. Remember that making her own mistakes is a guaranteed opportunity for her to learn very valuable lessons.

My mom has always let me make my own mistakes and I am now grateful for that. I can't go through life holding my mother's hand. My mom knew it was important for me to try some things on my own, and sometimes make a complete mess. It's from those messes that I learned the most. Mistakes are opportunities for us to learn how to get better at everything we do. As your daughter gets older, you have to learn how to let go while always being there for her as a safety net.

I'm now 17, and my mom has given me quite a bit of freedom. I have to tell her what I am doing and where I am going and if she is not comfortable with my plans, I have to change them. However, she trusts me to go where I say I'm going, and to do what I say I'm doing. There has to be trust between you and your daughter in order for your relationship to be secure.

Your daughter knows you love her, but make sure you tell her at least once a day. Every time my mom and I say goodbye, we always make sure the last thing we say to each other is "I love you". Once you and your daughter feel like you are both on the same team, you will have achieved a relationship that allows for honesty and openness.

Love,

Jordan

Q & A excerpt from our interviews with The Professional Health Team:

Girls Rock! **Teen:** What can moms do to set up habits of good communication with daughters?

Dr. Anne: Parents can be very reinforcing and supportive when daughters do open up about anything. Rather than reacting with any judgment or unwanted advice, tune into what they want from you and what they need to hear. Then balance it with parenting—communicating any concerns about their behavior.

Girls Rock! **Teen:** If girls and moms have difficulty communicating, how can moms initiate change?

Dr. Anne: Tell your daughter that you want a healthy relationship with her. Tell her how you are working on being a better listener—that you will stop judging or giving advice. You can go to therapy to work on your own skills. Invite her to talk at every opportunity, and pay close attention to any moment she does open up, and reinforce it as positive.

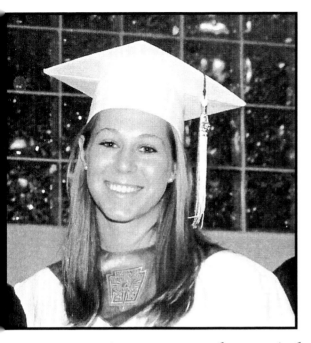

KIDS NEED CLEAR BOUNDARIES
Jenny Hafley, age 17

Dear Moms,

I remember the summer after 6th grade vividly. My mother and I were in a constant battle over my choice of clothing because she found it entirely inappropriate. It was the summer of the backless shirt trend.

My twelve year old self felt that this name— "backless"—was used for the sole purpose of scaring mothers because really, the shoelace-sized strip of fabric securing the shirt to the body, DID seem to constitute a back to the garment. Unfortunately for me (or so I thought at the time), my mother did not share this logic with me. We went around in circles about it. All I wanted to buy that summer was tiny revealing tops, but my mother felt I would be parading around in next to nothing.

She would not give in. I thought that this was the most unfair thing in the entire world. It seemed that if manufacturers were making shirts in my size, and clothing stores were advertising them to me, then they must be fine for me to wear.

That was almost six years ago, and clothing seems to have shrunk a little more every year since. I realize now that I was attracted to those swatches of fabric not just because they really were the only attractive options in the stores; I wanted to wear them because I knew they would draw attention. I saw models wearing them and looking gorgeous. The advertisements made it seem that the only way to happiness was through this minuscule clothing. I wanted to look grown up even though I was still just a girl.

Eventually, my mother allowed me to wear this backless-top thing to a party as long as I promised to keep a jacket on. It was a compromise I could live with, although I resented it and believed it was narrow-minded of my mother.

By the end of summer, it became clear to me that clothing would not change my life as I had previously suspected and dreamed it would. My lack of shirt-back at a party gained me no more friends, no more happiness, no more fun than I was already having as a pre-teen.

Now that I can wear whatever I choose, I no longer have the desire to wear the things I once did. I'm glad that my mom stood her ground with me and didn't allow me to follow through with a trend she knew wasn't good for me, even though everyone else was doing it. She was making the point that certain styles are damaging to young girls because they make them into women before being emotionally and physically ready.

I am guessing that you and your daughter will go through a similar experience. It may be a new clothing fad, or something else. Although I spent most of that summer fighting with my mom, I knew she was right.

Your daughter needs you to set limits and to stick with them. By standing her ground with me, my mom allowed me a little more time to just worry about being twelve. It turned out that I was having enough fun just as a protected girl with a shirt-back.

Love,

Jenny

Q & A excerpt from our interviews with The Professional Health Team:

Girls Rock! **Teen**: What do you most want moms to know about maintaining a healthy relationship together as a mom-daughter team?

Dr. Hood: Talking is really important. The questions I struggle with are, am I effectively communicating with my kids, and am I listening? I'm a working mother and I wonder if I am there enough. By us doing things together, hopefully we will not be just mom and daughters, but also friends. That's hard, too, because as the mother you still have to be the parent and the disciplinarian. But I want us to have a good interactive relationship. I think it's give and take.

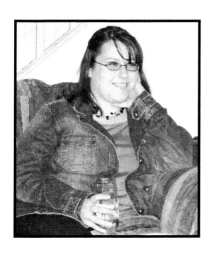

SPIRITUALITY AND BEING MY BEST SELF
Hillary Bullock, age 17

Dear Moms,

Oprah Winfrey said something in the February 2005 edition of her *O Magazine* that affected me. She said, "Now I live straight through the center of myself, which means telling the truth about everything. No more games. Every day I make the choice to live as well as I possibly can."

Beyond the many religions and traditions of our nation, I think that most of us try to practice our spirituality by living as sincerely as we possibly can. We want to be honest and moral and we want to try to help make a positive difference in the world. We want to grow up into strong, independent citizens who work hard to make positive contributions to society. This is why we become teachers, homemakers, athletes, ministers, social workers, and political leaders. We all want our lives to be a reflection of our beliefs and values — we want to be our best selves, and like Oprah, live as well as we can.

As I grow up, I struggle in coming to terms with the fact that my best self doesn't always match up with others' ideas of my best self. Society wants me to be "skinny" and rich, while some of my friends want me to be popular, but without crossing that line of being *too* sure of myself.

But I don't want any of those things for myself, and it has been a challenge to recognize what I do want in the face of those pressures. I have to ask myself about what makes me feel happy, secure, and confident. It has taken years for me to realize that happiness comes only when I focus less on what others want, and more on the constructive things I want.

For me, working with little kids, being involved with social justice projects, and expressing myself through the arts are crucial to my sense of who I am. I understand that beauty is not about the size of my clothes, color of my skin, or hairstyle. Instead, it's about all things sacred: creativity, my connection with a higher power, myself, and others.

Regardless of our diverse beliefs, most of us have a general idea of what our best self looks like: beautiful, creative, made for a purpose, generous, full of potential, loving, etc. When I immerse myself in these truths, I believe them!

Especially because girls and women are so pressured to focus on narrow beauty standards, it seems vital to teach pre-teens that beauty is about the light in them when they are doing something that they love. No matter their race, religion, or socio-economic background, every growing girl needs spiritual nourishment through constructive activities and perspectives.

And, like Oprah says about making a clear choice to live as well as she possibly can, girls of all ages can make good decisions for themselves when they realize they too have choices—and that while others' opinions can range from unhealthy to helpful, it is really one's own sense of best self that is most important.

I am happy to report that while I still struggle at times (like most of us!), I am striving to know what healthy things I do and don't want for myself, and I am using my right to choose between them. I want to hold my head high and walk with confidence. It has taken some time, but now at 17, the person I am reflects my best self more accurately.

Love,

Hillary

Q & A excerpt from our interviews with The Professional Health Team:

Girls Rock! **Teen**: Do you think spirituality is important for growing a healthy girl?

Dr. Griffith: I am a strong believer that one needs an inner balance or strength. My inner strength comes through my faith in God. Spirituality, however you define it, is important because no matter who you are, there will be times in life that require that strength. Unless you have something more, something deeper to ground you, you can be overcome and devastated. Faith is important.

Girls Rock! **Teen**: About faith, how do you nurture and replenish your spirit?

Dr. Griffith: I have a physical routine that I enjoy, I have moments when I read, and I like being around older members of the church because they represent such a tremendous source of strength.

TRANSCRIPTS

The following interviews were conducted by four of the authors of this book, with our professional health team, made up of experts from various fields.

Jordan Barnhill interviewed pediatrician Katrina Hood, Hillary Bullock interviewed pediatrician Joan Griffith, Jenny Hafley interviewed psychologist Anne Edwards, and Ravon Radmard interviewed dietician Donna Foster.

Jordan Barnhill's interview with pediatrician, Katrina Hood, M.D., F.A.A.P.

Jordan: You've been a part of the Girls Rock! *Team since the very first workshop in 2004—what made you want to be involved in the first place?*

Dr. Hood: At first, it was Lisa getting me involved. Her kids are my patients. I specifically remember the day, and I can even remember the room where we were sitting and talking. She said, "Hey I need your help, would you want to be involved in something like this?" She helped me understand where her kids were coming from with questions about all the stuff we incorporate within Girls Rock! workshops today, and then it really spurred my interest and made me think more about how I could make my physicals with kids here in the office more meaningful. So with all the ideas Lisa had, and with all of our discussions leading up to our first workshop, it is just amazing what we've accomplished for girls and moms in our community.

Jordan: Since focusing on healthy body image so much this past year, has your approach with your patients changed at all? How?

Dr. Hood: Drastically. Before, we had a set little thing we'd talk about: home, education, the activities they were involved in, drugs, sexual activity, and then you're supposed to talk about suicide as well. Now, since Girls Rock!, I incorporate more into my check-ups including: healthy eating, exercise, how they view themselves as people inside and out, feeling good about their body image, and then incorporating happiness as part of that. I really strive to make those four things come together for my patients.

You know people who are 100 years plus, they are healthy because they've realized how to stay healthy. I try to help my patients approach coming to see me as "How do I learn to be healthy right now? And what does it gain me?"

Jordan: At what age do girls begin to notice the changes of puberty in their bodies? What kinds of changes can they expect?

Dr. Hood: Generally, the earliest age is around 8 years old where some girls will have some breast development. I think mostly, you're looking at ages 9-11 as the usual ages when the breasts begin to develop. After the breast development comes the pubic hair and the darker hair on the legs. About a year or two after breast development come periods.

Jordan: How does weight gain figure into the changes that occur during puberty?

Dr. Hood: There is a healthy amount of fat that women need. It helps maintain regular menstrual cycles, a healthy body temperature, and a healthy heart. All girls at puberty will gain weight due to the effects of estrogen on fat cells in the body. All young women will have an increase in curviness of the hips, buttocks, belly, and breast. As long as a healthy body image and healthy foods are a part of their life, then they will be healthy.

Jordan: Should mothers talk to their daughters about these changes, and if so, what kind of information should they share with them?

Dr. Hood: My answer to that is that if a child asks a question, you give them just the information they asked for. So if they say, "Why do I have this little bump here?", you say "That's your breast developing". If they keep asking why questions, you keep answering. If you do it that way, you don't overwhelm them with information, and you can see what their natural curiosity is. But I always open the door in my check-ups with girls because a lot of times they are so embarrassed that they don't want to bring it up. So I try to tell them about the things that are coming so they will feel more comfortable talking to their own mothers about these issues.

Jordan: What is the one most important piece of advice you could give a mother about helping her daughter adjust to puberty?

Dr. Hood: I think that it is beautiful. So many girls are scared of it and they don't want to have the extra hair, the rolly tummies, or the curvy thighs, and bigger breasts. But all of that together makes you a woman. Seeing it as an opening of a window to the next part of your life is really exciting, and saying it's normal is important.

Also, having mothers talk to their daughters about what they went through and what they were concerned about would help. Talk about the different products you use for periods, so it's not embarrassing when it happens. It helps girls to be prepared if they happen to get their first period at school, so they aren't so scared. I believe that more knowledge is more power.

Jordan: Concerning your healthy body and spirit approach, are there certain things you often talk to your own girls about that you wouldn't mind sharing with our mom-daughter readers?

Dr. Hood: One of the biggest things we try to do is focus on being a family that does things together—being together, playing together, going outside to kick a ball around. I try to spend time every night with each one of my kids before they go to bed. I just ask them questions about the day or about things they want to talk about. It's a special time for them and me. I think that is important.

Most recently, my oldest daughter is excited about a little mom-daughter overnight we're going to take before school starts to talk about some of the puberty issues that will soon be coming up for her.

Jordan: What do you most want moms to know about maintaining a healthy relationship together as a mom-daughter team?

Dr. Hood: Talking is really important. The questions I struggle with are, am I effectively communicating with my kids, and am I listening. I'm a working mother and I wonder if I am there enough. By us doing things together, hopefully we will not just be mom and daughters, but also friends. That's hard too because as the mother you still have to be the parent and the disciplinarian. But I want us to have a good interactive relationship. I think it's give and take.

Jordan: From your experience in your practice as well as from mom/ daughter workshops, do girls tend to take after moms in how they feel about themselves?

Dr. Hood: Most kids adopt the patterns of their parents. So I tend to see healthy girls with healthy moms. If the mothers are making unhealthy diet choices and not exercising, then it is much easier for the child to make that choice. Ultimately, a family must take the path to good health together if a child is to make a lifelong choice for good health.

Jordan: What does "healthy spirit" mean to you personally?

Dr. Hood: A healthy spirit is what brings out a person's individuality—it is what makes each one of us different from any other. Each of us is on a journey to discover ourselves and to make healthy choices along the way—then we will have a healthy spirit.

Jordan: What advice do you give to your own daughters about being open-minded to everyone's differences?

Dr. Hood: When my girls ask questions that relate to differences in skin color, body type, religion and others, I first explain that it is natural for us to notice differences. How we react to those differences is ultimately what makes the distinction between acceptance of that difference and prejudice.

Jordan: Any final advice for girls and moms?

Dr. Hood: Televisions should not be in kids' rooms, and not in family rooms. Instead they should be behind doors in a room you have to go search out so it's not the focus of your home.

Also, I believe it's very important to have family meals together. It doesn't have to be a gourmet meal.

And, don't overbook your kids. Make their activities a part of their lives. Give them one or two things to be committed to, instead of running them around to countless activities that they have no time to focus on.

Parents should regain control and realize that they hold the power. They can monitor what their kids eat, do, and set healthy habits early.

Hillary Bullock's interview with pediatrician, Joan Griffith, M.D., M.H.A.

Hillary: What made you want to get involved with Girls Rock? Why are you passionate about this cause?

Dr. Griffith: I initially responded to an invitation to participate, and it felt very good to be involved. As a female with two daughters and two granddaughters, I think it's always encouraging to see families work together to make a difference—as well as have fun together. This is a great opportunity.

Hillary: What lessons do you like to share with the girls and moms who attend Girls Rock! workshops?

Dr. Griffith: I would like to think that the most important message I can share is that it is important to maintain balance in one's life—physically, spiritually, mentally, and emotionally. Once we maintain that balance, then life is worth living and enjoying.

Hillary: How do you define beauty?

Dr. Griffith: Beauty is that quality of life that makes you feel as if all's right with the world.

Hillary: Why do you feel that it's important for girls to grow up into healthy women?

Dr. Griffith: I think it's important that females realize that there is no better time than right now to be a female—to be energetic about life and the opportunities that avail—to be healthy and strong. I think health means that you have a positive attitude, even in the midst of trouble. It is important to be healthy in one's outlook so that you can survive the challenges of life.

Hillary: What roles do nutrition and exercise play in becoming a healthy adult?

Dr. Griffith: There's an old adage that we are what we eat. I think we are what we do, as well. Food is important because it keeps us nourished. Physical activity is important because it keeps us fit. When we are physically fit, we are often emotionally fit, as well.

Hillary: Do you think spirituality is important for growing a healthy girl?

Dr. Griffith: I am a strong believer that one needs an inner balance or strength. My inner strength comes through my faith in God. Spirituality, however you define it, is important because no matter who you are, there will be times in life that require that strength. Unless you have something more, something deeper to ground you, you can be overcome and devastated. Faith is important.

Hillary: Along the lines of faith, how do you nurture and replenish your spirit?

Dr. Griffith: I have a physical routine that I enjoy, I have moments when I read, and I like being around older members of the church because they represent such a tremendous source of strength.

Hillary: How do parents' habits with nutrition, exercise, and spirituality, affect growing girls?

Dr. Griffith: When we look at girls, I think one of the greatest influences can be a parent, especially a mother. Mothers are important because the food that is brought into the home, and the way food is prepared often centers around the mother. We recently completed a study that showed boys, as well as girls, are significantly influenced by the physical activity level of their parents, especially their mother. So I think mothers are critical, as we all know, in so many areas of life.

Hillary: Can you tell me about a woman who has made a great impact on your life?

Dr. Griffith: I can recognize several. If I think back to when I was a young girl in high school, the most significant person was my physical education teacher. She was energetic and sensitive, but I think the most important value she shared with me is that it is okay to dream and to try to achieve those dreams. As an older person, the most important lady in my life right now is the bishop of my church.

Hillary: Here's a million dollar question: If you could give one piece of advice to girls and/or moms, what would it be?

Dr. Griffith: Nurture your bond and rely on that bond to get you through the years ahead.

Hillary: It's great to be a girl growing up in North America today. How can moms help reinforce this to daughters?

Dr. Griffith: Mothers should first believe in their own hearts that it is okay to be a female, and then demonstrate that belief each day through actions and words. Their daughters will see it and emulate it. Daughters will not have to read about it, but will witness it in action each day—that is the most powerful teaching tool possible.

Hillary: How might moms help daughters create and achieve their own dreams?

Dr. Griffith: They can create a supportive, confidence-building atmosphere in which their daughters feel "it is okay to dream and even stumble so long as I get up and keep trying to be the best that I can be."

Hillary: Is there anything I haven't covered that you would like all of us to know?

Dr. Griffith: Continue to try to find a way to help girls realize it's okay to be a female. As a matter of fact, it is exciting to be a female.

Jenny Hafley's interview with psychologist, Anne Edwards, Psy.D.

Jenny: Why did you want to be involved with Girls Rock! ***in the first place?***

Dr. Anne: I wanted to become involved in Girls Rock! because I felt like it was a wonderful opportunity to educate the community about eating and body image concerns. I was very glad that it targeted girls and their mothers at a time prior to the likelihood of developing major problems in the hope of preventing them from occurring in the first place.

Jenny: Why is self-esteem important to empowerment in girls?

Dr. Anne: Self-esteem leads to empowerment because it is so hard to feel a sense of competence, motivation, and to take initiative without a healthy self-esteem. It seems like a cycle, that if you feel good about yourself, you feel more capable to explore your interests and succeed at them, which lead to you feeling good about yourself.

Early on, if you get in a negative cycle of feeling you are not going to succeed, or that you are not good enough to do something, it leads you to miss opportunities to show yourself that you are good at things. Sometimes you have to take chances, even if you don't think you'll succeed. You will likely feel proud that you tried, even if you aren't great at it.

Jenny: How important is mom/daughter time?

Dr. Anne: It is important for kids to have time with their parents to know that they have a solid base of support at home. It becomes very difficult for kids to figure out who they are and how they fit in with the world, but it can be easier to navigate if parents show support for them at home. Time together is the best way to show that you care.

Quality time should involve uninterrupted, non-distracted, periods of time with your kids. As far as how it is spent, it should be decided by the parents and kids. It can be doing something, or just taking a walk or sitting on a bench talking. The parent should be communicating that it is time set aside for the child because they care about her.

It is important for girls to know that they can communicate openly with parents, but they will not always opt to do so. They may see you as geeky or out of it and don't want your opinion. That is OK and normal. The most important thing is that she knows you are there for her and want her to talk to you and that any topic is acceptable. If you find that you do these things and your daughter doesn't communicate much with you, it can be helpful to offer for her to see a therapist so she knows that you care that she is heard by someone.

Jenny: What can moms do to set up habits of good communication with daughters?

Dr. Anne: Parents can be very reinforcing and supportive when daughters do open up about anything. Rather than reacting with any judgment or unwanted advice, tune into what they want from you and what they need to hear. Then balance it with parenting—communicating any concerns about their behavior

Jenny: If girls and moms have difficulty communicating, how can the moms initiate change?

Dr. Anne: Tell your daughter that you want it to change. Tell her how you are working on being a better listener—that you will stop judging or giving advice. You can go to therapy to work on your own skills. Invite her to talk at every opportunity, and pay close attention to any moment she does open up, and reinforce it as positive.

Jenny: Is physical exercise important to emotional health?

Dr. Anne: Research supports that exercise can affect your mood. The physical act of exercising releases chemicals that improve your mood. In addition, most people report a sense of pride or accomplishment by engaging in exercise. In addition, if it improves your physical health, your mood will likely improve as well.

Jenny: What is body image?

Dr. Anne: The definition of healthy body image is dependent on the culture. There are many cultures that don't assess or judge their bodies by appearance at all. In our culture, appearance is of such importance, that it is hard to determine what is healthy within such a culture.

I personally think that within our culture a healthy body image would include one of balance in which you feel good about how you look, what your body does, and that you spend the majority of your time focused on other concerns such as what kind of person you are, how you want to spend your time, who is important in your life, how your relationships are going, etc.

I believe a negative body image can take many forms with the balance of these factors being disrupted in some way. You may not like how you look. You may not focus on what your body does and only on how it looks. You may also tend to spend a lot of time focused on what you don't like about yourself and not much time on other important areas of your life. You may have a certain part of your body that you don't like. You may not like that you don't look like the girls on TV or in the magazines. There are many possibilities.

Jenny: How does peer pressure make us vulnerable to the influence of others?

Dr. Anne: Peer pressure is a typical part of growing up. Everyone wants to be liked and to fit in. As we mature, we try to figure out who we are and where we belong. This uncertainty leaves us vulnerable to others' influence. Others try to influence us to find their place in the world as well. When we are influenced to do things that don't feel good to us, we may be giving in to peer pressure.

Jenny: How is peer pressure affecting girls' nutrition today?

Dr. Anne: I hear a lot from clients about what happens during lunch at school. Girls seem to be very careful about what they eat. They also seem to be very vocal and judgmental about what others eat. Many people feel very self-conscious and don't eat a healthy meal like they normally would because all of their friends are only having a few chips for lunch. Girls also talk about their bodies and dieting which may make others feel that these things are and should be important to them, too.

Jenny: How does media affect a growing girl's sense of body image?

Dr. Anne: I think the media has a big impact on the culture as a whole, which puts an extraordinary amount of money into dieting and fashion and places little emphasis on inner beauty and other types of success. It is hard to live in a culture like this and make individual choices that differ from the overwhelming societal messages about what is important.

Jenny: How can parents send a positive message of health and nutrition to their girls in a diet obsessed culture?

Dr. Anne: Parents can help by communicating with their daughters how they have been impacted by the culture themselves, because we all have, and how they fight getting sucked into it. (Diets they have tried and the focus they have had on appearance and how now they are trying to simply eat healthy, balanced foods and focus more on other things.) They can connect with their girls by sharing this.

They can also make it a mission to fight the culture together. In the Girls Rock! workshops, I suggest to girls and moms to have some kind of code word that they can refer to when something catches their attention about negative eating or body image messages. For example, if a relative comments on your weight and you don't feel comfortable addressing it directly, you can look at your mom and use the code word to acknowledge that both of you know the comment is inappropriate and that you will discuss it later. The same word can be used when watching a commercial or walking by magazines in the grocery store.

Jenny: How can parents reinforce a positive self-image in their growing girls?

Dr. Anne: It is a difficult job, and you are not supported by our society. You have to seek out support to fight the cultural messages and instill healthy ideas in your daughter about her weight, eating, her body, and what is important in her life. The most important thing for you to do is to be a good role model. You must practice what you preach. If you are struggling, as these issues do impact all of us, helping yourself will be the best thing you can do for your daughter.

Jenny: What can girls do to build confidence in these transition years?

Dr. Anne: The way you feel about yourself will change as you grow and become a teenager and an adult. The best thing you can do to approach these changes is to build a solid positive self-esteem to carry you through the difficult times. Get involved in as many things as you can to improve your self-image. Talk to your mom and others when you question your worth. Talk to a counselor if needed.

Ravon Radmard's interview with dietician, Donna Foster, R.D., L.D.

Ravon: How did you first become interested in helping girls and women with their body image?

Donna: Well it came about as a result of my own issues with my body, my image, my eating disorders and through my healing. I wanted to bring this work to Kentucky because I didn't know of anybody who was really doing the work around food and healing body image.

Ravon: In your words, what is body image?

Donna: Body image is the picture you carry in your mind of what you look like. But there's so much more that goes into it than just coming up with an image. It starts in infancy with the way you're held and perceived—by the way our parents feel about us, how secure they are, because babies pick up on that. And then as you go on through your developmental years, how your mother feels about her body plays a very strong role in how we feel about our own bodies. So body image is made up not only of the mirror, but of our life experiences.

Ravon: What is an eating disorder?

Donna: An eating disorder is any way that one uses food to manipulate their weight, or a way a person copes with life in unnatural ways—denying hunger, eating when not hungry, any way that's manipulative of food.

Ravon: How do you feel about our culture's habit of weighing ourselves? How much should the numbers matter?

Donna: Not at all. How do you feel? Buy clothes that fit, that make you feel good! We don't need numbers. The more our culture is obsessed with thinness, and we have been, the bigger our population gets. And there is no acceptance of diversity in body sizes!

Ravon: Did you have role models who practiced healthy body image when you were younger?

Donna: No, my mother was uncomfortable with her body and she dieted. I remember getting into her dresser drawer, and there were candies called "ayds" used for dieting, and I would eat them because they were caramels, they tasted good.

Ravon: So how can Moms teach their daughters to love themselves physically?

Donna: By loving themselves first. And then it's automatically passed down.

Ravon: We hear the word "skinny" a lot in our culture, and a lot of time it's used as a compliment, what do you think about the use of this word?

Donna: I don't see that it's appropriate in any circumstance for someone to compliment with, "You are so skinny." That is labeling. I believe that it's inappropriate for anybody to comment on your body, or my body. It's a boundary violation, they're crossing over into something that they should not be making comments about.

Ravon: So what could be an alternative?

Donna: "You look beautiful in that color," or "You look great today, really put together." "Looks like you feel good, or have good energy." Or, "That outfit is so flattering on you." But not about size. What gives another person the right to comment on size? If someone says something to me about my body—and it doesn't happen anymore, but it used to—I feel invaded, scrutinized.

Ravon: In your opinion, what is the cause of girls not having healthy body image in our country?

Donna: I think the culture is certainly involved, but we're into third-generation eating disorders, so it does go back to mothers, and grandmothers. It's so deep and until we start exploring the depths of a woman, and she is willing to go deeper than what she looks like, it won't change.

Ravon: About third-generation eating disorders, do you see a lot of girls suffering because of something said by a family member?

Donna: Oh, yes. There's something called a "One Comment Syndrome". This is most common in girls or boys at the age of middle school, and one single comment is said and they're off and running. You know from being children in elementary school and not really being conscious of your body to all of a sudden changing in one year and being self-conscious of your body because of those changes, and getting interested in the opposite sex. Then somebody makes a comment and the child feels overly self-conscious.

Ravon: It's like the domino effect?

Donna: Very much so, ONE COMMENT. Other kids have the build-up of comments over years. Parents are terrified that their child will be "fat", and they impose restrictive health practices or eating behaviors in themselves around the image of being healthy.

Ravon: So where is the line crossed by a parent who wants their child to eat healthy but who is afraid of their child becoming "fat" or overweight?

Donna: The line is crossed when the amount of time and attention becomes more than it should be, and when it's really emphasized, and that's the only thing the child hears. It's a balance. It's normal for bodies to change throughout a person's lifetime, and if parents are okay with their bodies, their children will see that.

Ravon: Who are the people in the media that you view as healthy role models for young girls today?

Donna: Jamie Lee Curtis is someone I really admire. You know, she has girls, and I think she's terrific! She allowed *Vogue* magazine to photograph her without any touch-ups in a bathing suit, and she has a woman's body. And Emme is another great role model. And Oprah is—everyone has watched her process, she's not perfect, nobody is, and she's still had to do the work on becoming healthy. I think she's an excellent role model for women about what women can do no matter what their background.

Ravon: A lot of people believe that "healthy food" means low calorie food. What does it really mean to eat "healthy"?

Donna: Eating healthy is choosing primarily from the main food groups, real food. In a healthy diet there is room for fun foods, treat foods. But when that becomes the mainstay of your diet, it becomes unhealthy. There are choices even in fast food that are healthy.

We've gotten away from family meals and eating at home, and it's a terrific challenge in our culture to eat healthy because we are presented with unhealthy food choices everywhere.

Ravon: What's an example of something healthy found in an everyday fast food place?

Donna: There are some really good salads in all of them—and grilled chicken instead of hamburgers—fruit and yogurt parfaits. You can order scrambled eggs and an English muffin at McDonalds and have a perfectly adequate breakfast! You can get small portions instead of the oversized portions typically served. Get a hamburger but don't get fries; add a side salad. There are many options, but I don't see people doing it.

Ravon: How old is your granddaughter, and what kind of guidance do you give her about healthy choices and lifestyles?

Donna: My oldest granddaughter is 11, and the day she was born, I thought: This is a real cross-roads for me, I am going to mentor this girl in this toxic society. And the best way to do that is to achieve my own personal goals in my life. There are a lot of great books for children on body image. And talk about feelings! All feelings are OK. Allow girls to have a voice!

I took her when she was 9 to a play that UK [University of Kentucky] put on for eating disorder awareness week called *What's Eating Katie?* and afterwards I asked her, "What did you get out of that, Emma?" and she said, "If you get that voice in your head about not being good enough, then ignore it!" That's it, she knows!

I maintain an open dialogue with her.   If girls are talking about weight and bringing it out in the open, she's going to be OK.

Ravon: Do you believe there is a spiritual component to health?

Donna: Completely. At the root of all the pain is a spiritual starting. It's an emptiness, a void, a sense of not being complete. Being alone, and having to maneuver live without adequate skills instead of having something more powerful than your own ego there to assist you.

Ravon: What would you say to struggling mothers?

Donna: Do your own work. Get help because you are molding your daughters. There is hope out there, and, even though it's a small movement, it's an important movement, and the people out there, Jamie Lee Curtis, Emme, Oprah, and Lisa with *Girls Rock!*, provide hope!

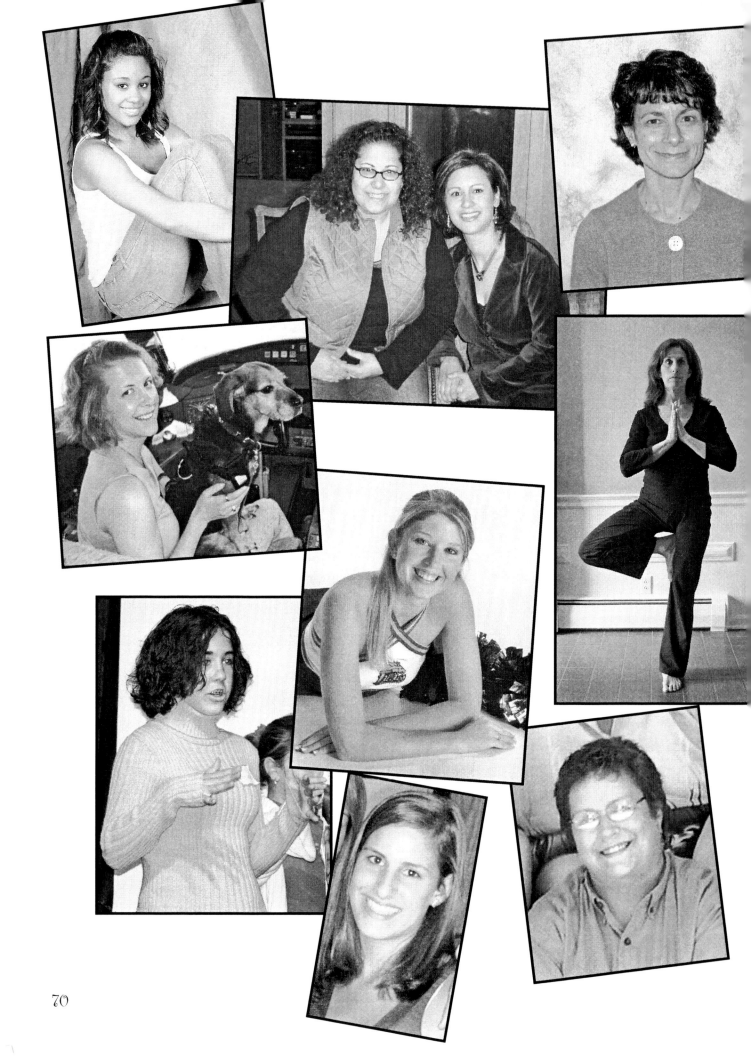

Afterword for Girls and Moms

TO MY FUTURE DAUGHTER
Jasmine French, age 15

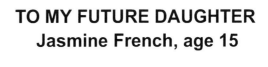

Dear Daughter,

Being the teenage girl that I am now and knowing what it's like growing up makes me want only the best for you. I can already feel it, you're going to be beautiful no matter what. Be the beautiful girl God is making you!

I want you to be healthy: take care of your body, eat good foods, and exercise. I want you to find things that you love to do. Maybe you will take after me and cheer, or be involved in church with youth group and ushering.

I love music like R&B and gospel. I love being outdoors, especially in spring and summer, riding my bike, just hanging out, and walking in the park. Maybe these things will bring you happiness, too.

I will teach you to believe in yourself. Having confidence and keeping your head high is called self-esteem. All people need self-esteem to manage challenging times and it might be hard, but we all get through it. Like my mom says to me today, "Always listen to me and you'll be okay!"

You should know that making mistakes is good because you learn from them, and become smarter and stronger. No matter your mistakes, I will always love you and I will always have your back.

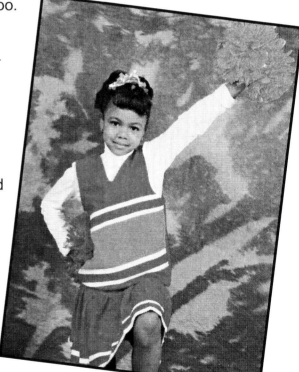

me at age 9

Choose good role models and by watching them, you will know how to be strong. Today, Queen Latifah is a woman who accepts herself no matter what, and she is an inspiration to me. You will be inspired by someone, too.

I want you to live your life to the fullest each day and have fun! It's great to be a girl and to have girlfriends. You get to have sleepovers with late-night talks, go to movies and the mall, and do all kinds of stuff that girls love to do together. Choose friends who believe in you and who want the best for you. Be a good friend to others.

Being a girl can sometimes be hard. I tell myself all the time that I don't want you to have to go through the same stuff I did. From peer pressure to struggling with self-esteem, growing up isn't always easy. But you know, that is just part of it all. We all get through it. I will always help you.

Try your best to be a good leader and know that it's also okay to be a follower as long as you are doing what's right. For both, think about working hard, staying focused, and listening to others' suggestions.

There are some specific things I want for you, like going to a good college to get a good education. Make good grades and try to be your best so you can accomplish your dreams. I want you to be who you want to be. Be yourself!

When you have a family, raise your kids well. Help make them be just as wonderful as you are. Do the same thing for your daughter that I'm doing for you now—write her a letter and let her know that you are always there.

To be all of this—strong, smart, happy, living your dreams—you must believe in yourself. Don't let people pressure you into doing things you are against or that you don't believe in! I want you always to do what you know in your heart is right.

Most importantly, I want you to talk to me about anything and everything—your fears, worries, questions, and concerns. I will always be here! Don't ever feel like you can't talk to me. Mother/daughter conversations are the best ones. Right now, I know that my mother is here for me and she is one of the strongest things that keeps me going. Without her, I'd always be looking for a guide. So, know that I'm here, and never hold anything back.

I love you.

Love,

Your Future Mother (currently age 15)

Q & A excerpt from our interviews
with The Professional Health Team:

Girls Rock! **Teen**: It's great to be a girl growing up in North America today. How can moms help reinforce this to daughters?

Dr. Griffith: Mothers should first believe in their own hearts that it is okay to be a female, and then demonstrate that belief each day through actions and words. Their daughters will see it and emulate it. Daughters will not have to read about it but will witness it in action each day. That is the most powerful teaching tool possible.

Girls Rock! **Teen**: How might moms help daughters create and achieve their own dreams?

Dr. Griffith: They can create a supportive, confidence-building atmosphere in which their daughters feel, "it is okay to dream and even stumble so long as I get up and keep trying to be the best that I can be."

"GRATITUDE" ACTIVITY

Gratitude is a powerful force which helps to sustain feelings of inner peace and which actually helps to attract positive influences to us. Also, by dwelling in gratitude, we wire our bodies and minds to embrace goodness—the sweet little things in life that can mean so much every day.

Like a magnet, your feelings of gratitude will draw to you opportunities for your own fulfilling future.

There are tiny miracles everywhere waiting to be noticed and enjoyed by you. Together, explore what this means and, using the space below, list all the things in your lives that you are grateful for right now. You may consider creating a family gratitude journal in which you regularly record your feelings of gratitude. It will be fun and interesting to realize what your loved ones appreciate.

MOMS

I feel grateful for...

GIRLS

I feel grateful for...

Resources: Recommended Books, Magazines, and Websites

For Moms and Dads

Daughter's Newsletter: For Parents of Girls, www.Daughters.com

Real Kids Come In All Sizes: 10 Essential Lessons to Build Your Child's Body Esteem, Kathy Kater

Renewal: A Time for You, Deepak Chopra and Women First Health Care

Reviving Ophelia: Saving The Selves of Adolescent Girls, Mary Pipher

When Women Stop Hating Their Bodies, Jane Hirschmann

Women's Bodies Women's Wisdom, Christiane Northrop, M.D.

www.DadsAndDaughters.org
> This organization teaches dads how to thrive as compassionate advocates for their daughters.

www.EatRight.org
> The American Dietetic Association provides valuable food and nutrition resources.

www.NationalEatingDisorders.org
> The National Eating Disorders Association provides resources for prevention and intervention, including treatment referrals.

www.StirItUpAmerica.com
> The Stir It Up Campaign encourages parents to join together in improving kids' nutrition in school, family, and community.

www.TheCompassionateCommunity.com/GirlsRock/
> The Girls Rock! website provides additional information and a link to purchase more copies of this book.

Classroom Curriculum

Full Mouse, Empty Mouse, A Five Day Curriculum, Dina Zeckhausen, Ph.D. (www.edin-ga.org)

Healthy Body Image: Teaching Kids to Eat and Love Their Bodies Too, Kathy Kater (www.NationalEatingDisorders.org)

Nurturing Girl Power: Integrating Eating Disorder Prevention/Intervention Skills into Your Practice, Sandra Friedman (www.NationalEatingDisorders.org)

For Girls and Moms Together

The Care and Keeping of You: The Body Book for Girls, Valorie Lee Schaefer & American Girl Library

Chicken Soup for the Girl's Soul, Jack Canfield, Mark Hansen, Patty Hansen, Irene Dunlap

New Moon: The Magazine for Girls and Their Dreams, New Moon Publishing www.NewMoon.org

www.GirlsOnTheRun.org
> Girls on the Run is a non-profit prevention program that encourages preteen girls to develop self-respect and healthy lifestyles through running.

www.GirlScouts.org
> Girl Scouts of the USA provides an accepting and nurturing environment in which girls build character and skills for success in the real world.

www.MindOnTheMedia.org
> Mind on the Media seeks to expand the definition of beauty, raises public awareness about depictions of girls and women, offers free media literacy action kits, and hosts the annual "Turn Beauty Inside Out" conference.

www.YMCA.net
> Across the nation, local YMCA community centers promote individual and family fitness, including team sports. Ys are welcoming for all people of all faiths, races, ages, abilities and incomes.

www.YWCA.org
> The YWCA provides safe places for women and girls, builds strong women leaders, and advocates for women's rights and civil rights in Congress.

Lexington Herald-Leader, June 15, 2004, page D1.
Reprinted with permission.

Get fit Kentucky

'Girls Rock' teaches a realistic outlook

Workshop covers nutrition, self-esteem, portrayal of women in media

By Sara Cunningham
HERALD-LEADER STAFF WRITER

As Lisa Miller worked in her home office a few months ago, she heard her two young daughters talking just outside her window about something that surprised her — they were talking about being fat and being thin.

Miller said she had always made it a point to avoid using such words as *fat* and *thin*. She showed the girls pictures of women with average body shapes who are famous for their beauty, and she talked to them about health, Miller said.

"I knew I was already doing everything I could at home to help my girls get positive, realistic body images," Miller said, "but it was still happening."

That's when Miller decided to do more. In two months, she created a curriculum to help combat the negative messages about what women should look like.

Her workshop "Girls Rock: Self-Esteem, Healthy Body Image and Empowerment" this month at Temple Adath Israel brought Miller's ideas to fruition.

It is one step in an effort to shed light on the many influences that affect our images of health and beauty.

See IMAGE, D8

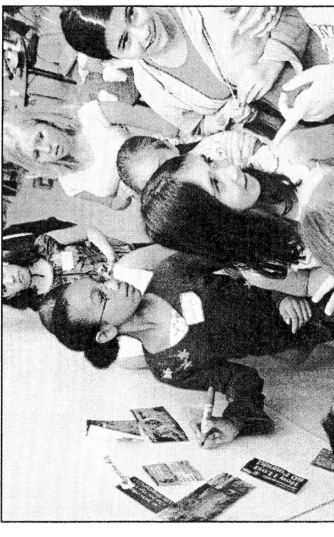

BRIAN TIETZ

Sofie Tapia, left, Emily Miller, foreground, both of Lexington, and other girls described how images of women in the media make them feel during "Girls Rock" on June 6.

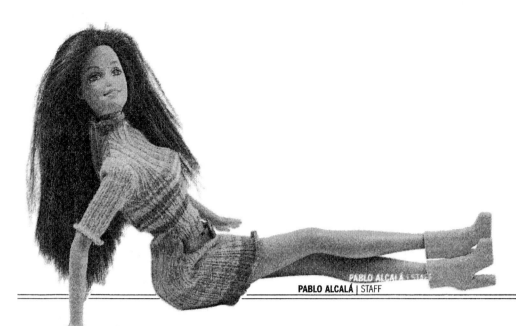

PABLO ALCALÁ | STAFF

IMAGE | Eliminate the word 'diet,' pediatrician says

From Page D1

About 15 mothers and their daughters, ages 8 to 13, joined Miller and her two daughters, 8 and 10, as they listened to doctors, police officers, self-defense instructors and others talk about health, self-esteem, nutrition, body image and the media.

Psychologist Ann Edwards said the way mothers talk can have a huge effect on the way daughters think.

"Even though they'll deny it," she said, "they pay attention to what you listen to, what you say, what you eat."

One of the hot topics for both generations is nutrition and dieting.

Pediatrician Katrina Hood told the group that the word "diet" shouldn't even be in their vocabulary.

"At some point, a diet comes to an end — and then what are you going to do?" Hood said. "This should be about learning to make healthy decisions as a family, for every member of the family. It is a long-term lifestyle change."

A big obstacle mothers and daughters face is that even if they go to a workshop and make changes, other relatives or friends might make negative

More information

In putting together packets for mothers to take home from the "Girls Rock" workshop, Lisa Miller included excerpts or samples from the following resources:

■ "Daughters," a newsletter for parents of girls. You can subscribe to it, or get more information at www.daughters.com.

■ *Your Dieting Daughter: Is She Dying for Attention?* by Carolyn Costin (Brunner/Mazel Trade, $25.95).

■ *When Women Stop Hating Their Bodies* by Jane Hirschman and Carol Munter (Ballantine Books, $14.95).

■ *Hunger Pains* by May Pipher (Ballantine Books, $12).

■ *The Wonder of Girls* by Michael Gurian (Atria Books, $14).

■ *You Have to Say I'm Pretty, You're My Mother* by Stephanie Pierson and Phyllis Cohen. (Simon & Schuster, $23).

■ *When Girls Feel Fat* by Sandra Friedman (Firefly Books, $14.95).

■ *101 Ways to Help Your Daughter Love Her Body* by Brenda Lane Richardson and Elane Rehr (Quill, $13).

■ *Unbearable Weight* by Susan Bordo (University of California Press, $4.70).

---

comments, Edwards said. It's hard, she said, to educate everyone at the same time.

"It's so hard because you work to give your daughter a positive example, but who knows what a grandmother, uncle or family friend will say in front of her?" Edwards said.

Edwards recommends that mothers and daughters come up with secret signals or codes to use with each other when those things happen. She said

that no matter what progress mothers and daughters make, a comment from another family member such as "you look like you've lost weight" or "you look chunkier" can still hurt.

A simple wink or nudge from an understanding mother can remind the daughter what's really important without hurting the feelings of the other family member, she said.

"Just some private way to connect with your daughter as

if to say, 'I know it's not OK, and you know it's not OK, and we'll talk about it together later,'" she said. "It will keep that connection."

Carol Kaplan, who attended the workshop, said she is interested in anything that helps her teach her kids how to make healthy choices.

Her daughter Katie, 12, said she had a class and school assembly where students learned about healthy choices and healthy body images, but it wasn't enough. Her mother agreed: "It should be a whole lifetime of learning."

Reach Sara Cunningham at (859) 231-1443 or 1-800-950-6397, Ext. 1443, or scunningham@herald-leader.com.

MEET THE AUTHORS!

KATIE ATKINSON, AGE 16

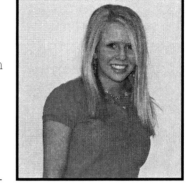

Hi I'm Katie Atkinson. I'm a junior in high school. I like to read and travel, hang out with my friends, and spend time with my family. At school I'm involved in being a DARE (Drug Abuse Resistance and Education) role model—I talk to younger students about staying drug free.

It's important to me to be a role model to younger kids. Through DARE I help students to be positive and healthy in making decisions because there are lots of influences out there, so we all need someone to look up to. Through Girls Rock! I enjoy helping younger girls who are about to go through the same things I experienced.

Also, because of being born with out a left arm, I have had to fight being labeled as "different". I have overcome many challenges with the way I feel about myself. Today, I enjoy expressing myself about my experiences so that other girls can find encouragement. I hope you all take some wisdom and insight from this book.

KATHERINE BANDOROFF, AGE 16

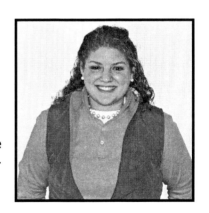

I am Katherine Bandoroff. I am 16 years old and a sophomore in high school. I have a younger brother and sister. Although we push each others' buttons, my brother Conrad is very proud of my athletic achievements and is one of my biggest fans. My sister Isabel is ten years younger than I am, and we have a very close relationship. I see myself as a second mother to her, and I know that she is always looking up to me. My parents own a horse farm where they breed, raise and sell horses.

Throughout my life I have never been "skinny"; I am a broad-shouldered and muscular girl, and I do not have a problem with this. I am an athlete, and I am happy with myself because this is who I am.

Sports are a major part of my life. If I'm not at school, I am either at practice or working out to improve my performance and strength. I am very determined, and I work extremely hard to accomplish my goals. As I think about my future, I hope to be playing soccer in college while majoring in sports medicine.

I am involved in writing this book because I know I am a good role model. Many girls question their body image and question who they are. This can cause a loss of confidence. I know I can help because I have succeeded in the activities I love, and I want to make it known to all girls that if you believe in yourself and love yourself, you can accomplish anything you want in your life.

My goal for this book is to make people aware that looks are NOT part of what makes up a good or a healthy human. I also hope that you mothers and daughters can strengthen your relationship by discussing the issues we introduce.

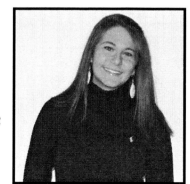

JORDAN BARNHILL, AGE 17

Hi! My name is Jordan Barnhill. I am 17 years old, and I will be a senior in high school. I am an only child and have a dog named Oliver. I love the theater and have been active in plays since I was a little girl. I love to see movies, go on vacations, and hang out with my friends.

I am so excited to be a part of this book. Most media images portray picture perfect bodies, faces, and clothes. They can cause us to feel less important because we do not look the same way. This book provided me with an outlet to express my opinions about these unobtainable images. It shows girls and moms that it is possible and important to be happy with ourselves as we are. Once you are content with yourself, everything else will fall into place. I hope you enjoy this book, and most of all, I hope it helps!

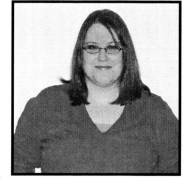

HILLARY BULLOCK, AGE 17

Hey! My name is Hillary Bullock and I am a 17-year-old junior in high school. Growing up as the middle child has given me a unique perspective in life.

My parents have always emphasized the importance of education, and while that is important, my creative activities (playing piano, flute, creative writing, making jewelry, decorating my room) are what really make me happy. I also really enjoy falling into a good book, being around kids, and sleeping in on lazy Saturday afternoons. These are joys I wouldn't give up for the world!

Having attended public schools my entire life, I've learned quite a bit about other people and their cultures. This exposure has instilled in me awareness, respect, and appreciation for the similarities and differences of people within my community. Gaining an even deeper understanding of others is important to me; it is the reason I plan to major in social work in college. For the time being however, I am very active in school, community, and church activities.

Another reason I'm passionate about Girls Rock! is because I learned the hard way that without a strong sense of myself, it was impossible to create any kind of balance in my day-to-day life. For many years, I did not make the best decisions regarding my physical, mental, and spiritual/emotional health. The road was long and hard, but I'm a better person because of it and am thrilled at the opportunity to pass my wisdom along to you.

JASMINE FRENCH, AGE 15

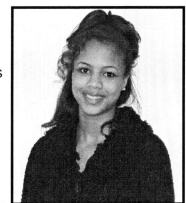

Hi, I'm Jasmine French. I'm a sophomore in high school. I'm on the cheerleading team and have been cheering since I was 7 years old. I'm in the Student Council, and Harambee club at my school (African-American cultural activities). I also like acting and public speaking. During my freshmen year of high school I took drama, a class that gave me a taste of theatre. I really enjoyed it and I plan to explore this more once cheerleading season is over.

I've been learning Spanish since first grade and am now fluent. My dream is to be a Spanish Interpreter for the FBI.

I enjoy being a Girls Rock! mentor because it's a beautiful thing, and I believe in helping girls feel good about themselves.

Girls, It's important that you know that everyone goes through changes and that you are not alone. Change helps us become strong which gives us self-esteem.

Hopefully by reading this book, you will get a better understanding of life itself, see what other girls just like you have been through, and learn how they've dealt with it to become strong!

JENNY HAFLEY, AGE 17

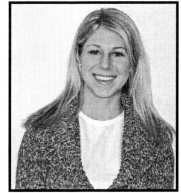

Hi, my name is Jenny Hafley. I am a 17-year-old senior in high school. As you will probably come to find, I really enjoy talking about issues that I consider important; one of those is the empowerment of young girls.

I am a busy person, and I love being involved in activities that motivate and inspire me. I am active in school organizations, but am most active in programs outside of school that address diversity issues in our country. For that reason, my participation in both the Mayor's Youth Council and Camp Anytown, are very important to me. In my free time I love to read, go to concerts, take pictures, draw, travel, play softball, and hang out with my friends.

I cannot believe that I have the opportunity to help write a book about something I am so passionate about. I feel so fortunate to know the amazing group of girls and women that make up our Girls Rock! team. Together, we are sharing with you something we have felt in our hearts for a long time. These are all the things we wished someone had shared with us when we were your age.

For example, I wish someone outside of my family had made it clear that no matter what a girl looks like, she is beautiful—and that with effort, I can be anything I want to be. I wish I had been told that the size of my body and the shape of my stomach should not matter to others, and that it's the compassion in my heart and the strength of my convictions that count more than anything else ever will.

It's my hope that as you continue to read this book, you will think of us as your friends and companions. It is awesome to be a girl growing up today! We are excited for you, and we are offering some wisdom since we have been where you are now!

I hope you enjoy this book as much as we enjoyed creating it for you!

ABBY MILLER, AGE 9

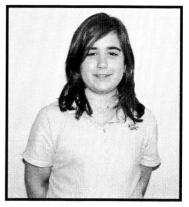

My name is Abigail Miller. I'm 9 years old. I'm in fourth grade, and I'm an animal lover. I have a sister, a mom and a dad, and a dog named Apple, and I love them very much. I spend most of my time reading, drawing, and playing outside.

I'm excited to be a part of this book because I like helping other people. Also, I don't think it's fair that some people think that girls shouldn't do stuff that boys do.

Moms and girls should read this together. It's good for both of you because you will spend time together and learn together about a lot of things that are good to know about growing up.

Hope you enjoy it!

EMILY MILLER, AGE 11

Hey, my name is Emily Miller. I am 11 years old and in sixth grade. I like to play basketball and softball. I enjoy watching Kentucky basketball with my dad, and I like hanging out with my mom. I love to act and perform. I love my Jewish overnight summer camp, and I like to be outside with my friends.

I wanted to help with this book because I think it's important for girls and women not to judge each other on how they look, but to appreciate the beauty inside. People focus too much on how to stay thin instead of loving themselves and enjoying their lives.

I think it's important for you to read this book because you will learn that beauty on the inside is more important than just beauty on the outside. After reading it you will have a whole new positive attitude about your body. This project has helped me and I hope it helps you! Enjoy!

CHAUNCEY MORTON, AGE 15

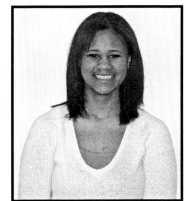

Hey, I'm Chauncey Morton. I'm 15 years old, a sophomore in high school, and one of 6 children. I am an optimistic person, easy to talk to, and I always consider others' opinions. I enjoy hanging out with my friends and just being myself. In my community I'm involved in the Youth News Team, Lexington Youth Leadership Academy, and the Mayor's Youth Council.

I decided to become a Girls Rock! Teen Mentor because I enjoy being a role model and I feel this is a way for younger girls to connect with older girls in a positive, healthy way. The programming provides a wonderful way for younger girls to ask older girls about issues they are experiencing.

I hope that you are able to take something valuable from this wonderful book that we have all come up with.

RAVON RADMARD, AGE 17

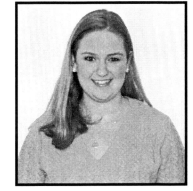

My name is Ravon Radmard. I am seventeen years old, and attend The School for the Creative and Performing Arts. I am in the student council, Beta Club, the Principal's Forum, and am editor of our literary magazine. I'm involved in church and the Mayor's Youth Council. I plan to go to college next fall, and I hope some day to pursue a career in medicine.

Outside of all that, I am just a teenage girl who like many, has been struggling with weight and body image issues for many years. I am tired of my friends, family, and the media, telling me that I need to look thin and perfect. After all, what is perfect? My long-lasting happiness does not come from reading a bathroom scale or the size of a sweater—but this is not what I've been led to believe from childhood to adolescence.

I have found that my happiness comes from unconditional love, activism, creative writing, spirituality, and doing a good job in the projects I commit to. Out of all my extra curricular activities, being able to work as a teen mentor in promoting healthy body image for younger girls has been one of my most rewarding experiences.

I hope that with this book, girls and moms will redefine beauty. I hope it excites you about your individuality. I hope that this book helps forge an even stronger bond between you.

MOLLY GALLAGHER SYKES, AGE 18

Hi, my name is Molly Sykes, and I am going to be a freshman in college. I just graduated from high school, and I'm 18. I'm contributing to this special project because I had a hard time when I was growing up as an adolescent girl and I wish I had had a book like this. Adolescence can be a trying time and girls need support before they get there.

I have participated in Girls Rock! as well as Mayor's Youth Council, the Lexington Youth Leadership Academy, and the Global Youth Leadership Conference. I've always been a girl who wants to go the distance, and my inspiration during my teen years came from my mother. That's why I want to reach out to mothers, too.

I love to read and write, draw, ride horses, and be active in any way I can. I'm a perfection-ist all around, and some adults mistakenly look upon me as the 'perfect child'. However, I have had problems and faults just like any other girl; but I was able to deal with them in a positive manner through support from loved ones and professional help. My greatest hurdle was anorexia nervosa, a deadly eating disorder.

I hope that this book helps each reader gain some insight—mothers and girls alike. We all need support, so, go on and take it! Read these stories and advice, and discuss them together.

MEET THE PROFESSIONAL HEALTH TEAM

Anne L. Edwards, Psy.D.

I have four kids: a 13-year-old stepdaughter, and two year-old triplets—one girl and two boys. I am a psychologist in private practice. I enjoy anything outdoors—hiking, camping, laying under the stars, reading, and drawing, though I mainly change diapers and watch Elmo right now.

As an eating disorder expert, I spend a lot of time listening to women who don't like how they look, how much they weigh, who they are.... I am very excited and proud to be part of a project that is emphasizing the positive in being girls and women, and helping others to do the same.

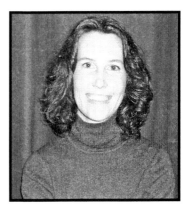

859-229-6753

Donna Foster, R.D., L.D.

I am the owner of the Kentucky Center for Eating and Weight Disorders. I run some of the nutrition and wellness group sessions offered, as well as private nutrition counseling sessions. My hobbies are: family including grandkids, reading, home.

I'm excited to be part of this project mentoring young girls to overcome the pressures of a toxic culture, in order to grow into confident young women who are comfortable in their own bodies.

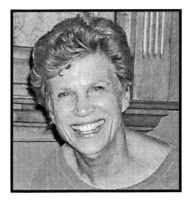

859-219-8953
www.kcewd.com

Joan Griffith, M.H.A., M.D.

I retired from the Air Force after 21 years of active duty service. I have been a pediatrician here at the University of Kentucky for approximately two years. My biggest job here at UK is working with the TEAMS Clinic (Teens Enjoying Active Management Systems) to help children who are overweight develop better eating and physical activity habits, as well as improved self-image.

For me, involvement in *Girls Rock!* and this book provides an exciting opportunity to help shape the future generation.

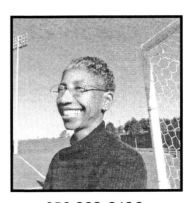

859-323-6426

Katrina Hood, M.D., F.A.A.P.

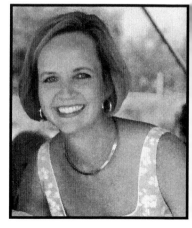

After medical school, I served in the U.S Navy for seven years. My husband and I have three children, who are between the ages of five and ten years old. I'm a full time pediatrician with Pediatric and Adolescent Associates, and I serve as Chair of the Department of Children's Services at Central Baptist Hospital.

I've been a part of Girls Rock! since its inception. As a pediatrician, I see so many young girls worrying about the external instead of the internal. Being a part of this team project has helped me communicate to girls about what is most important.

859-277-6102
www.paalex.com

Lisa Miller, Mother of tween girls, Founder and Chair of Girls Rock! Healthy Body Image, Self-Esteem, and Empowerment Workshops for Pre-Teen Girls and Moms.

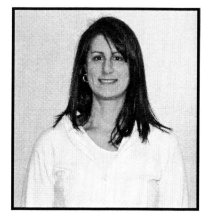

I grew up in Canada and now live with my husband and two daughters in Lexington, KY. I'm a full-time mom and part-time everything else, although Girls Rock! projects do get a lot of nurturing! I love family gatherings, reading, everything about the outdoors, and many kinds of crafting. And chocolate.

It has been a pleasure to work on this project, which brings together the strong voices of so many girls and women. I love the message that we are all okay, and I love that my daughters feel it. Girls really do rock just the way we are—this is a valuable message to live by.

GirlsRockKY@aol.com